Melasma
…is this the clear solu

By

Vanessa Wild

This book is also available in e-book format, details of which
are available at
www.authorsonline.co.uk

An AuthorsOnLine Book

Published by Authors OnLine Ltd 2002

Copyright © Authors OnLine Ltd

Text Copyright © Vanessa Wild

The front cover design of this book is produced by Jane Brownhill, Chris Ruffles and Vanessa Wild ©

The moral right of the author has been asserted

All rights reserved. No part of this publication may be reproduced, stored in a retrieval system, or transmitted in any form or by any means, electronic, mechanical, photocopy, recording or otherwise, without prior written permission of the copyright owner. Nor can it be circulated in any form of binding or cover other than that in which it is published and without similar condition including this condition being imposed on a subsequent purchaser.

ISBN 0 7552 0062 4

Authors OnLine Ltd
15-17 Maidenhead Street
Hertford SG14 1DW
England

Visit us online at www.authorsonline.co.uk

About the author

My name is Vanessa Wild, a.k.a. Ness. I am a busy self-taught artist and mother with no medical credentials to my name. I have always had an avid interest in alternative therapy and have educated myself on the benefits of nutrients for many illnesses and conditions on an at-home basis over the last ten years.

For three of those years I suffered from melasma, which was partly brought about, I believe, by the over-use of prescription drugs. Having always been a staunch believer in the benefits of alternative and nutritional therapy and, like many others, having had no luck with any of the conventional methods of treatment available, I set about finding a 'cure' for this aesthetically-embarrassing and demoralising skin disease. By pure chance and luck, I happened upon a remarkable nutrient called MSM Sulphur, and realised the therapeutic benefits it offered this particularly stubborn condition. Consequently, I have shared my views and personal opinions, with regards MSM treatment for melasma, with more than 100 sufferers worldwide, of all ages and races, many of whom are now well on the road to recovery.

I intend, despite any possible negative criticism that the information provided within may incite, to continue to spread the MSM word via this book in order to help many others who find themselves desperate for an alternative and safe solution for the treatment of melasma, a disease that has, so far, eluded a cure. *That* is my sole and honourable intention behind writing this book. I am, in no way, associated with the sale, distribution or profits of MSM Sulphur.

I wish you all luck and happiness in your potential recovery.

Acknowledgements

This book would not have been possible without the support and co-operation of all those who, free-willingly and bravely, took part in my experiment which was conducted via the Internet over many months. A special thank you goes out to each and every one of you for displaying courage, sharing your heartache and joy and detailing your experiences of this MSM Sulphur therapy via your messages throughout the trial. I am indebted to your faith in my natural therapy beliefs, and despite the fact that this treatment may not work for everyone; together we have, and hopefully will continue to gradually bring a smile back onto the faces of many others who are in despair of ever being able to face the sun again.

Thanks especially to Mel for the sound and witty literary advice and to V. Lam for setting up the 'Melasma Family' Community. Thank you to all my friends from the 'Melasma Family' who provided unfailing encouragement and support; you know who you are.

Thank you to Baz, Nic, Chris and Jane, at Mirashade Ltd for being there throughout whenever I needed assistance with my book, whether it was for proof reading, cover design skills or just for an ear to bend!

Thanks goes to Jane Iredale for kindly providing product information, makeup tips and general support.

Special thanks also goes to Dr. Stanley W. Jacob, MD, of the Oregon Health Sciences University in Portland Oregon, Robert Herschler, a research scientist for Crown Zellerbach, for all their years of research on MSM. Both Dr Jacob and Robert Herschler share in the patent and marketing rights to MSM.

Also thanks to Dr. Ronald M. Lawrence MD, PhD, and Martin Zucker, a health writer, for all their own research carried out on MSM.

To my twin sister, Justine, for her fantastic editorial support - thank you!

Last, but not least, love and thanks to David for being my rock – I couldn't have done this without you.

Disclaimer

My book features the details of an ongoing experiment that involves the use of a nutrient called MSM Sulphur for the therapeutic treatment of melasma. Beyond what is anecdotal or hypothetical, there are many well-known facts featured within this book regarding both melasma and MSM independently of one another. The MSM therapy, as set out in my book, must be undertaken entirely of your own free will.

You acknowledge and agree that, by reading the contents of this book and method of treatment herein, choosing to undergo this self-treatment is your own decision and at your own risk and that this therapy and any information contained in or provided through this book is provided on an "as is" basis. N.B. The information in this book has not been scientifically or professionally investigated or proven, nor has it been evaluated by the Food and Drug Administration or any other agencies and no minimum or maximum daily requirement of MSM has yet been established.

You understand and agree that the information contained in or provided through this book is intended for general consumer understanding and education only and is not intended to be and is not a substitute for professional medical advice. Always seek the advice of your dermatologist, physician, nurse or other qualified health care provider before supplementing with MSM and for answers to any questions you may have generally regarding MSM or any existing medical condition prior to embarking on this therapy. Nothing contained in or provided through this book is intended to be or is to be used for medical diagnosis or treatment.

Under no circumstances whatsoever, including, but not limited to negligence, shall I or any other parties mentioned within this book, be liable for any direct, indirect, special, incidental or consequential damages, arising out of the use, or the inability to use, the materials, treatments or therapies published within this book.

This book is dedicated to David and George

authors OnLine

Melasma
…is this the clear solution?

by

Vanessa Wild

Contents

What is Melasma?	1
Risks and Potential Causative Factors	3
Current Treatments Available	9
Makeup	13
My Story	17
MSM Sulphur	27
MSM: Is this the Clear Solution for Melasma?	30
Questions and Answers	32
Testimonials	49
Abbreviations	102
Glossary	103
References	107
Recommended Reading	108

1

What is Melasma?

Melasma, or chloasma as it is also known, is a very common disorder of cutaneous hyperpigmentation and is commonly known as 'the mask of pregnancy'. It is the formation of irregular-shaped brown spots or patches of varying shades on both sides of the face, especially on the forehead, nose, cheeks, upper lip, chin and on other sun-exposed areas of the body. An increase in tyrosinase activity in the melanocytes found in the epidermis of the skin is a major factor in the development of these patches, and coupled with sun exposure, thereby yields an increase in melanin production. The distribution of the three most common kinds of melasma (centrofacial, malar and mandibular) is usually symmetrical and can be referred to as dermal or epidermal in type, with dermal melasma being the most stubborn type to treat. It is capable of spreading over time if left untreated.

A dermatologist can identify what type of melasma is present, i.e. dermal or epidermal, by means of a Wood's Lamp or Light. Epidermal pigment is enhanced during examination of the skin under the ultraviolet light emitted, whereas dermal is not. A large amount of dermal melanin will be suspected if the hyperpigmentation is blue-black in colour. Dermatologists can treat epidermal melasma successfully using some of the treatments currently available (see Current Treatments Available chapter).

Unfortunately, dermal melasma is much more difficult to treat, and using the same methods of treatment as those used for epidermal melasma can yield unpredictable results. It is thought, however, that if epidermal melanogenesis can be safely inhibited for long enough periods of time, then dermal pigment (where tyrosinase activity is not present, hence the non or little response to topical therapies available) will not replenish and could slowly resolve and normalise over time. Commonly, sufferers have both types of melasma present.

Melasma is predominantly observed in expectant or menopausal women and in those taking oral contraception or hormone replacement therapy. This could be the reason why the most commonly believed causative factor is a hormonal imbalance or fluctuation that can render the skin more susceptible to developing darker patches of pigment, particularly when exposed to sunlight and regardless of the use of a high factor sunscreen. However, melasma can occur independently of these hormonal factors, can even affect some men and unnervingly, seems to be increasingly commonplace in all ages and races worldwide.

Above all, melasma is an extremely distressing condition for all those who develop it, and many feel dismayed at the lack of sympathy, support, care and attention given during professional consultations. Inevitably, those who suffer lead a more sheltered life because the patches can darken spontaneously whilst undertaking outdoor activities, thus creating a phenomenal negative impact on their social lives.

Until now, I did not believe that a safe and effective therapy even existed for the treatment of stubborn dermal pigment.

Risks and Potential Causative Factors

Hormonal changes or fluctuations during pregnancy and the menopause or during use of oral contraception and hormone replacement therapy (HRT) can all play a role in the development of this condition, making the skin more susceptible to developing dark patches of pigment when exposed to sunlight. Oestrogen, progesterone, and melanocyte-stimulating hormone (MSH) are normally increased during the third trimester of pregnancy. In some cases the pigment can fade after pregnancy and the menopause, or after discontinuing use of oral contraception and HRT, but in other cases the pigment remains steadfast and help is required.

A genetic predisposition tends to be a major factor in the development of melasma and certain skin types seem to be more prone. Human complexions are generally classified into the following six skin types:

- Type I - light skinned, burns easily, never tans.

- Type II - light skinned, burns easily, tans a little.

- Type III - light skinned, burns occasionally, tans well.

- Type IV - light skinned, tans well, rarely burns.

- Type V - brown skinned (e.g. Asian, Indo-Asian, Chinese and Japanese), tans well, rarely burns unless exposed to ultraviolet radiation for prolonged periods.

- Type VI - black skinned (Afro-Caribbean), deeply pigmented, very rarely burns, even after prolonged exposure to ultraviolet radiation.

The higher the skin type, i.e. types IV and up that tan easily, therefore tend to be more susceptible to developing the condition, but paler skin types can be affected as well, particularly if living in regions of the world where there is intense sun exposure.

Ultraviolet radiation can cause peroxidation of lipids in cellular membranes, leading to the generation of free radicals, which could over-stimulate the activity of the melanocytes causing the production of excess melanin. Even incidental exposure, such as indoor strip lighting, the home fire, computer terminals, UVA rays from sunlight permeating car windows, and other heat sources are thought to be able to aggravate melasma.

However, self-induced trauma to sensitive skin types, e.g. waxing of facial hair (especially of the upper lip and even plucking eyebrows), chemical exposure, allergic reactions to skincare products or other types of skin inflammation, can all precipitate or exacerbate the condition.

Personally, I believe that mild Adrenal Insufficiency or Adrenal Exhaustion can play a role in the onset of melasma. Adrenal Insufficiency is a condition where the adrenal glands (situated immediately above the kidneys) are compromised in their production of cortisol and other steroid hormones, collectively known as corticosteroids. Primary symptoms can include:

• Fatigue

• Confusion

• Anxiety or panic attacks

• Impaired memory

- Low motivation or lethargy

- Apathy

- Weakness

- Decreased appetite with ensuing weight loss

- Nausea, possible vomiting

- Abdominal pain

- Diarrhoea or constipation (which could be misdiagnosed as Leaky Gut Syndrome or Irritable Bowel Syndrome)

- Abnormal pigmentation of the skin

Additionally, those with mild Adrenal Insufficiency tend to have an increased susceptibility to all kinds of infections including those caused by bacteria, viruses, parasites, yeast, and fungi.

Chronic Adrenal Insufficiency (very low or no corticosteroids) produces a more serious condition called Addison's disease, which produces similar symptoms to those mentioned above. However, these symptoms are generally more extreme in nature, e.g. anorexia and extensive pigmentation of the skin including the gums (inner mouth).

Adrenal Exhaustion or Low Adrenal Function is observed when the body has been subjected to prolonged stress. This stress could be caused by infections, exposure to toxins or chemicals, sleep deprivation, nutritional deficiencies, the loss of love or emotional support and hectic lifestyles. The adrenal cortex (outer covering of the adrenal glands) produces corticosteroids to increase blood sugar levels for this resistance reaction to stress. This response is in order to sustain energy and elevate blood pressure and an overuse by the body's defence mechanism in this phase could eventually lead to disease. Blood sugar levels also decrease over time as the adrenals become depleted and this, in turn, can lead to a decrease in stress tolerance and progressive worsening of mental and physical exhaustion, and possibly illness.

Typical primary symptoms of Adrenal Exhaustion could include:

• Fatigue

• Inability to recover from exercise

• Muscle and joint pain

• Irritability

• Depression or low self-esteem

• Insomnia

• Headaches

• Increased allergies

No matter the reasons behind them, the unfortunate but typical reaction to emotionally stressful situations is to indulge in high sugar 'comfort' foods, turn to stimulants such as caffeine (i.e. coffee, tea or cola) and nicotine, drink excess alcohol or even take recreational drugs. Inevitably, all these factors would weigh heavily on the already-weakened adrenal glands' ability to function well.

A high protein and low fat diet, as well as yo-yo dieting, crash diets, drastic weight loss treatments and even regular eating 'on the run' can also have a negative impact on the adrenals.

Any of the above factors could easily affect the delicate endocrine system in the process thereby further increasing the risk of developing or exacerbating melasma.

Other possible predisposing factors that contribute to the development of melasma, in my opinion, are:

• Naturally-existing hormonal irregularities, e.g. ovarian disorders.

• Nutritional deficiencies, especially B-group vitamins, caused by a poor diet (e.g. consuming pre-packaged or 'junk' food), or poor internal health (e.g. Leaky Gut Syndrome, Irritable Bowel Syndrome or Candida Albicans) that can affect proper assimilation of dietary nutrients.

• A poor immune system or sluggish liver function.

• Other existing health factors or problems e.g. thyroid disorders.

• The intake, especially if taken on a regular basis, of specialist photosensitising prescription drugs, e.g. allergy or acne medication.

• Living in highly polluted parts of the world.

• The consumption of food and drink containing high levels of additives, pesticides or chemicals.

• A build up in the body of a cocktail of chemicals from years of toiletry product use, e.g. shampoos, deodorants, perfumes, hairsprays, bath and body products, that can eventually be stored in the fat cells, tissues and organs of the body and consequently disrupt the endocrine system in both men and women.

In all of the above cases, and where melasma has been formally diagnosed by a physician or dermatologist, avoiding the sun, wearing a hat, and applying a broad-spectrum, high factor sunscreen is of paramount importance.

Sunscreens are agents that physically or chemically block the penetration of UV light into the skin. Sunscreens usually contain more than one agent to provide greater protection and those that provide protection from both UVA and UVB waves are called full or broad-spectrum sunscreens. Just using sunscreens that block primarily UVB radiation alone will be unreliable, as longer wavelengths will also stimulate melanocytes to produce melanin.

When used as directed, a sunscreen rated SPF 15 is usually adequate for most skin types, but those with an SPF greater than 15 may be even more protective but unfortunately, are more expensive. Because they contain multiple sunscreen agents in higher concentrations, they can also increase the risk of irritation and the development of contact allergies, which in turn can increase the likelihood of pigmentation developing. It is therefore advisable to avoid products containing chemical sunscreen agents such as PABA (B-vitamin para-aminobenzoic acid), cinnamates, benzophenone and oxybenzone, which are known to cause allergies. Products containing the less irritating, physical barrier-type sunscreen agents, namely titanium dioxide and zinc oxide, that physically form a barrier between the skin and the sun by reflecting or scattering the sun's rays, are much safer for use by melasma sufferers. However, it is worth knowing that adverse effects to sunscreens are, on the whole, relatively uncommon.

Current Treatments Available

Many treatments for melasma and other forms of hyperpigmentation (such as post-inflammatory hyperpigmentation, for instance, following cutaneous trauma arising from injury or inflammatory diseases such as acne), are currently available in the form of 'quick fixes' with destructive modalities, e.g. cryotherapy, chemical peels and lasers. Many practitioners attempt to speed up the recovery process with the use of mild exfoliation by means of microdermabrasion techniques or superficial chemical peels using, for instance, glycolic acid. They rationalise that with a high keratinocyte turnover coupled with the application of bleaching agents like hydroquinone to arrest melanogenesis, the recovery time will be shortened. These techniques, however, have proved to produce unpredictable results for some sufferers.

Epidermal melasma or superficial hyperpigmentation may, in some cases, respond favourably to any of the methods of treatment outlined below. However, dermal melasma rarely responds to these same treatments that can, in some cases, even exacerbate it, induce post-inflammatory hyperpigmentation and increase photosensitivity instead. It would therefore be advisable to consult a dermatologist who can ascertain what type of melasma is present before embarking on any of these treatments:

Hydroquinone:
Hydroquinone inhibits melanogenesis. It is available in a cream, gel or solution formula and can be found in various 2% strength over-the-counter products or obtained via prescription only at a strength of 4% plus. Hydroquinone produces variable depigmentation results. Prolonged topical use of some products containing hydroquinone can promote

permanent loss of pigment (hypopigmentation) within the hyperpigmented macules or, where concentrations used are higher than 5%, may cause a paradoxical hyperpigmentation, also considered permanent and untreatable. As a result, high-strength hydroquinone is generally prescribed for short periods of time only.

Another major problem, commonly encountered with this treatment, is the failure to apply the hydroquinone-based product precisely to the macules themselves. This would, inevitably, lighten the surrounding unaffected areas of the skin in the process and would leave the skin with varying degrees of hypo and hyperpigmentation.

Topical Tretinoin:
Topical 0.01-0.1% tretinoin can be effective in the treatment of superficial facial melasma but may take up to 24 weeks for any clinical improvement. Topical tretinoin may cause transient stinging and it can produce some erythema and peeling. Photosensitivity may also occur. Tretinoin is available in a cream or gel base or as a solution.

Hydroquinone & Tretinoin in Combination:
Available as a solution or in a gel or cream base, hydroquinone combined with tretinoin can fade melasma more rapidly and efficiently than topical hydroquinone alone. The same side effects that are produced by these two ingredients individually can be observed.

Glycolic Acid:
Glycolic acid (an alpha hydroxy acid or AHA) is used as a chemical peel. AHAs have been used to treat some superficial forms of melasma and the treatment involves a series of peels in progressive concentrations. For better results, it is recommended that AHAs be used in combination with hydroquinone and high factor sunscreens. AHAs can cause transient, mild stinging and in higher concentrations used for

peeling, erythema may also develop, which generally lasts for only a few days. Scarring, hyperpigmentation and hypopigmentation are also possible reactions. Experience of the therapeutic potential of AHAs in melasma treatment is still evolving.

Azelaic Acid:
Azelaic acid has been shown to be effective in treating some forms of hyperpigmentation. A possible explanation for the efficacy of azelaic acid in the treatment of melasma is related to its selective effects on hyperactive melanocytes. Azelaic acid generally inhibits the activity of tyrosinase and the most commonly reported adverse symptoms are transient stinging and itching.

Due to azelaic acid being, largely, a particularly effective treatment for epidermal melasma or some forms of superficial hyperpigmentation, with little cause for concern regarding side effects when compared to hydroquinone, this is often the dermatologist's treatment of choice.

The use of topical steroids, such as hydrocortisone, as a single depigmenting agent to treat melasma is generally not encouraged as there is always the possibility of inducing secondary skin conditions such as acne rosacea, perioral dermatitis or other types of inflammatory diseases.

With all of the above treatments, complete sun avoidance and continuous application of sunscreens are critically important for good results. Unfortunately, it must be borne in mind that, for dermal melasma sufferers in particular, even a minimal amount of sun exposure can instantly undo any progress made with the above treatments.

No matter whether the melasma is severe or not, camouflage makeup is useful in helping the sufferer to recover any lost self-esteem and confidence. It is advisable to use a good brand of makeup that contains a high SPF as well as one that is effective at concealing the affected areas. The next chapter covers my personal recommendations for makeup.

4

Makeup

Makeup. Where would we be without it? It is one of our staunchest allies in our battle against melasma. However, finding a good brand that camouflages the macules effectively without looking too caked and theatrical is difficult and usually costs a small fortune in our quest to find the right shade and coverage, not to mention the fact that the chosen brand must provide protection from the sun as well.

Many of us who suffer from melasma, are eager to bridge the gap between embarrassment and confidence in dealing with this morale-crushing condition, and therefore would welcome a few good tips on makeup products that contain safe lightening agents and sunscreens.

One such makeup brand name, in my opinion, fits the bill perfectly - Jane Iredale. These products are truly outstanding and rate highly in all the necessary criteria expected in a good choice of makeup for all melasma sufferers.

Jane's lovely products contain a highly sophisticated blend of minerals and pigments that are micro-pulverised, using proprietary technology and processes to form microscopic flat crystals. These crystals overlap each other on the skin to form a filter that allows the skin to breathe and function normally while still protecting it from air-borne pollutants. The staying power of the minerals is so great that they rarely need a touch-up during the day. And because these silky-feeling powders are water resistant, they won't crease or smear even during the most strenuous exercise. The water-resistant factor is also a true bonus for all those who are afraid to go swimming or even get caught in a downpour for fear of their makeup washing off.

Most importantly, the bases provide full protection from both UVA and UVB rays because the safe, physical sun-blocking ingredients, namely titanium dioxide and zinc oxide, act like mirrors on the skin.

Jane's range includes loose and pressed mineral powder bases called 'Amazing Base® Loose Mineral Powder Base' and 'PurePressed® Compressed Mineral Powder Base' respectively. The pressed base provides an SPF of 17, the loose, an SPF of 20 and both are a concealer, foundation, powder and sunblock in one. The bases, available in a range of ten different colours, can be applied to clean skin after moisturiser has been absorbed and can be used wet or dry. There is no need to use any other concealer or foundation whatsoever, therefore cutting down the time taken to conceal and blend in the macules every morning, a task that can in itself be an arduous and tedious one. Your choice of base colour would depend on your needs; for example, if you need to conceal redness after laser or chemical peel therapy, then a yellow-toned base will suffice. If you need to just conceal the macules, then choose a tone that closely matches your overall complexion. If necessary, two base colours can even be mixed together to gain the most suitable, corrective coverage. Because the minerals reflect light, they have a much wider tolerance than most makeup.

Here is a breakdown of what these amazing bases can do for you. They:

• Come in such a large range of colours that there is one for every complexion, no matter what the ethnicity

• Contain no fillers

• Pose virtually no allergy risk

• Are composed of inert materials that cannot support bacteria

- Are anti-inflammatory and help to calm other skin conditions e.g. rosacea, dermatitis and acne

- Contain minerals that heal and nourish the skin during use

- Are non-greasy/non-comedogenic (will not block pores)

- Are easy to apply

- Cover well, even after laser resurfacing and chemical peels

- Are natural looking

- Stay put all day long with minimum need for touch-ups

- Protect the skin from pollution

- Contain a broad-spectrum (both UVA and UVB) high SPF using safe ingredients

- Are very water resistant (rating by an approved FDA lab)

- Are environmentally aware and not tested on animals

Jane Iredale also developed the first global mineral base colours for her 'Global Shades' range. There are eight lovely shades ranging from deep gold to deep mahogany and they were created to suit skins and nationalities as diverse as African American, Asian, Hispanic and European. The exclusive formula of these PurePressed global bases also provides a foundation, powder, concealer and sunscreen all in one and replaces the need for liquid and cream foundation. They are formulated to control oil and provide unsurpassed coverage and staying power. The PurePressed bases also contain titanium dioxide and zinc oxide, pine bark extract, which is a potent topical anti-oxidant, and jojoba ester, which improves skin texture and reduces moisture loss.

For any extra and necessary coverage, or for those 'barely made-up' days that we all crave when you don't wish to apply full-facial makeup, Jane has a product called 'CoverCare™ oil-free cream'. This soft concealer can effectively conceal hyperpigmented macules, birthmarks, scarring or small amounts of redness or bruising after surgery. Loose mineral powder may be mixed with CoverCare and then thinned with moisturiser in order to change the colour. When it dries, it will stay put on the skin until removed with cleanser. The mineral powders may be applied over the top of CoverCare if desired.

A recent addition to Jane's range is 'Enlighten Concealer™'. This product contains three very safe lightening ingredients: Licorice, Vitamin K and Arbutin. Arbutin is a new state-of-the-art ingredient from the bearberry leaf that checks the formation of melanin by inhibiting tyrosinase activity. Arbutin is a very safe and non-toxic skin agent that does not have the potential side effects of hydroquinone. It has been especially developed to not only conceal, but help lighten hyperpigmentation of all kinds as well.

The Jane Iredale range, also known as The Skin Care Makeup, is so safe and beneficial to use that it is recommended by plastic surgeons and dermatologists throughout the world. For more information about Jane's amazing range, including the countries her products are sold in, you can visit her website at **www.janeiredale.com**.

So, now that you know how you can safely and effectively conceal melasma and boost your self-esteem, read on to discover how I came upon, potentially, your most important ally in your battle against melasma: MSM.

My Story

My name is Vanessa Wild, otherwise known as Ness. I am not a qualified GP or nutritional therapist, nor do I have a PhD in science or any other such qualification to my name. I have, however, studied Food and Nutritional Science as part of an Hotel Management and Catering course at Manchester Polytechnic, UK, in 1988. Due to a naturally keen interest, I continued to study the topic of nutrients and educated myself on their benefits for many conditions and illnesses on an at-home basis over the ensuing years.

I have always wholeheartedly believed in the merits of orthodox medicine in general, but, suspicious of the growing impact on my personal health of many prescription drugs, such as antibiotics, given throughout the Nineties for minor, common ailments, I understandably began to develop an aversion to them. Following treatment with most of these drugs, my diagnosed conditions tended to recur with a vengeance and metamorphose into yet another problem after a short period of remission, leading me down the never-ending road of ill health, both physically and emotionally. These problems took the form of:

• Recurrent candidal infections, e.g. thrush, a fungal toe-nail infection and Tinea Versicolor

• Urinary Tract Infections

• Irritable Bowel Syndrome

• Suspected Leaky Gut Syndrome

• Food intolerances

- Fatigue

- A scan-proven swollen ovary

- Endometriosis

- Menstrual irregularities

- Blood sugar imbalance/sweet food cravings

- Other inflammatory skin conditions such as Perioral Dermatitis

- Depression/irritability/dizzy spells

In a vain attempt to do something about my declining health, from time to time, I would enthusiastically embark on a few self-imposed or professionally recommended alternative health programs in an attempt to remedy some of my conditions. But unfortunately, despite believing that alternative treatment would be best course of action for me in my quest for improved health, being weak-willed, I failed to resolutely adhere to all but one program due to my hectic lifestyle. In some cases, my resolve failed due to the unwelcome detoxification side effects (such as nausea and headaches) that I inevitably had to endure in order to feel well again. However, I did manage to introduce probably the singularly most important health program of all; I started to drink at least 1 litre of water a day in 1999, which did partially relieve the symptoms of some of my conditions, particularly those of IBS.

In the same year, after taking a strong drug, albeit reluctantly, prescribed to 'cure' yet another problem that arose, small patches of pigmentation appeared literally overnight on the central parts of my face. I didn't make the connection to this particular drug at the time and I wasn't even taking any form of oral contraception. Thankfully, the macules would pale along with my growing concern and virtually disappear throughout the winter months. But, to my utter horror, they would return the following summer alongside new patches that would appear on even more sun-exposed areas of my face, such as my forehead. This trend continued for three years, during which, left unchecked due to my ignorance, the macules grew larger and spread progressively.

Eventually, curiosity got the better of me and I began to fully educate myself on what I suffered from. I discovered that I had a common skin disease called melasma, and I read numerous articles on the possible causes of the condition and available treatments. These treatments, all of which I tried and tested, included off-the-shelf skin-lightening products, prescription-only topical creams, yellow light laser therapy, microdermabrasion, and even, out of sheer desperation, acupuncture. Every single treatment failed to clear the macules permanently and, in some cases, worsened my condition. Disillusioned and depressed, I finally succumbed to booking an appointment with a private dermatologist in order to avoid waiting a further six months for treatment on the NHS waiting list.

The dermatologist took one minute of my time and £90 of my money to diagnose what I already suspected that I had. I was shattered to learn there really was no known singular cause or cure. I was curtly informed that I probably had a genetic propensity to acquiring the disease, given a prescription for a strong bleaching cream, advised to stay out of the sun and told to "get on with my life". I cried hard on my way home as the horror dawned on me that I would have to live with these permanent 'tattoos' on my face and never be able to look at the sun with confidence again. Dreams of long, exotic holidays and carefree outdoor activities and pursuits evaporated in the face of this stark reality. Despite the tears, that day turned my life around as I vowed with steely determination to find an effective therapy for melasma if nobody else could help me.

My research had me delving deep into the dusty recesses of every library and bookstore, only to be dismayed to find that there truly were no answers to this seemingly incurable disease. My attention turned to the World Wide Web, the so-called Information Super-Highway, to see if that at least could provide me with some clue as to how to get rid of my melasma. Nothing. Only treatments producing temporary results seemed to be available, many of which tended to work for epidermal melasma, but not for the dermal, more stubborn type of melasma that I suspected I had. I couldn't understand why so little research had gone into the underlying causes of this unsightly disease, a condition that seemed to be so prevalent worldwide, with 6 million sufferers in the USA alone.

Desperate for answers, luck came about in the form of an Internet chat room specially developed for fellow sufferers. After reading all the posted threads, the answer leaped out at me from every cry for help. I noticed that practically all the female participants of the chat room had taken prescription drugs in some way, shape or form. Birth control pills, antibiotics, specialist drugs and even steroid inhalers seemed, in my eyes, to be capable of precipitating the onset of melasma. Many of us shared common illnesses as well, that the very same drugs could have induced, and even more alarmingly, not everybody was taking or ever had taken the birth control pill or any other synthetic hormone-based drug, which were the most commonly presumed causative factors. It dawned on me that all the expensive topical therapies available were not producing the desired depigmenting effect in most of the participants, many of whom also seemed to suffer from dermal melasma, because this was a condition, I believed, that clearly needed to be tackled from inside the body itself.

I began to spend all my spare time researching ways on how to help encourage the body to heal itself, from the inside out. I surmised that, for some of us, the immune system needed a helping hand and targeting the possible poor health of the organs was key, particularly the adrenals, liver and gut, that the drugs could have had a detrimental impact upon. If liver spots could occur on the hands and faces of aged people whose immune systems and organ function were naturally failing due to the ageing process and in whom nutritional deficiencies were likely, then could the various drugs we had all taken have had a similar, maybe severe, impact on our organs, for instance the gut, thereby impairing its function? In other words, could the drugs have promoted an imbalance of intestinal flora, thus inducing digestive disorders, nutritional deficiencies and symptoms and a gradual decline in health? Furthermore, could the drugs have had a severe impact on our delicate endocrine systems that govern our hormones and their respective levels? That is, could they have had a debilitating effect on our adrenal glands thereby inducing hyperpigmentation commonly observed in those suffering from mild or chronic Adrenal Insufficiency?

Guesswork aside, and determined to tackle, once and for all, my other aforementioned long-standing health problems that I had failed to treat successfully using prescribed orthodox treatments, I continued my research via the Web. Almost certain by now that they were drug-induced, I suspected that my additional health problems were somehow interrelated with the development of my melasma. After much research, I chanced upon an article about the general benefits of supplementing with pure MSM Sulphur; it seemed, at least, to be the answer to all my other problems. I learned that it had hormone and pH balancing properties that help to eradicate acidic-pH-thriving pathogens like Candida Albicans. MSM was capable of soothing and healing the lining of the gut thus improving food intolerances, allergies, digestion and the consequent proper uptake and assimilation of nutrients, many of which I seemed to have a deficiency in. Reported as being an all-round immune system booster to boot, and despite potentially producing negligible side effects such as those common to the detoxification process, e.g. mild headaches and nausea, I decided to take the plunge and practically ran to the health store to buy it.

I felt the benefits of taking MSM overnight, literally. My energy levels soared, mental alertness improved, my hormones and blood sugar levels stabilised and I felt a sense of wellbeing and emotional calm that I hadn't experienced in years. Even the side effects from the detoxification process were very short-lived and alleviated by drinking plenty of water, to which I had, of course, become accustomed. Three days later, I made to wipe what I thought was a blob of cream from my forehead patch of melasma. It didn't move. On closer inspection, I realised that the 'blob' was a crack revealing normal-coloured skin. Over the next few days, many more appeared, some joining together to form larger gaps. I excitedly informed the women from the Internet chat room of my findings, whereupon many decided, of their own free will, to follow suit and, to my amazement and joy, many of these women also began to experience this strange and wonderful phenomenon.

As the number of participants grew on a daily basis, I began to collect statistical data and feedback over a 6-month period from approximately 100 women who had decided to try MSM. All of the women, some of whom contacted me privately in order to maintain their privacy, suffered from stubborn facial melasma that ranged from mild to extensive that had been unresponsive to conventional treatments.

Within 6 months:

• 60% of those who had tried MSM had positive results, albeit to varying degrees (see some of the feedback kindly given in my Testimonials chapter).

• A further 15%, many of whom had just embarked on the treatment, so it was too early to ascertain whether MSM was working for them or not, were still waiting to observe changes.

• 9% thought that they could see minor changes e.g. some breakup and/or overall lightening, but needed more time to be certain.

• 5% found that they were hypersensitive to MSM or simply couldn't tolerate the uncommon, minor side effects such as headaches and mild abdominal cramps, and gave up on the therapy. Some of these women, unfortunately, held jobs that did not enable them to drink plenty of water throughout the day which would have helped them to overcome these symptoms.

• 1% suffered from an allergy to sulpha drugs, and despite being aware that MSM was a different and safe kind of sulphur, decided not to proceed.

• Initially, 10% of the women were disappointed to observe no changes at all despite their best efforts to ascertain what factors could be hindering their progress. However, during the time taken to write this book, it transpired that of these 10%, a few of the women did eventually observe changes after either a long wait of 3-4 months and/or when having increased their dosage considerably to a level that they still felt comfortable taking. Therefore, it proved to be fortunate that they had persisted with the MSM program either through sheer determination, or because they enjoyed experiencing the other positive effects of taking MSM.

Overall, the time taken to see results varied from 12 hours to 4 months plus. It is difficult as yet to determine why the discrepancy is so large, however, a few of my personal theories are outlined in my Questions and Answers chapter.

To date, I know of no other therapy for stubborn, dermal melasma, natural or orthodox, that has yielded such a high percentage of positive results. At the time of this book going to print - a total of 7 months into the MSM experiment - the approximate number of women experiencing positive results to varying degrees was nearing 100. The exact number of women who have recovered, and still are recovering, might never truly be known due to the unknown number of women who could have happened upon the chat room experiment, tried out the MSM therapy, chosen to remain anonymous and therefore not actively participated in any of the feedback. As such, statistically speaking, the recovery results could indeed be much higher than those stated above. My chapter on testimonials features feedback regarding the changes that were observed periodically throughout the first 6 months of my MSM experiment by some, not all, of the women who took, and still are taking part. All the women's testimonials, which also include the additional benefits gained from taking MSM, were kindly given to myself with their express permission.

On a more personal level, the additional benefits that I was thrilled to experience after a few months of MSM supplementation included the following:

- My skin instantly turned very soft overall, my eyes brightened, my hair grew thicker and glossier and my nails strengthened. My circulation improved and I developed warm feet for the first time in years!

- All my fungal conditions vanished including the stubborn toenail infection that had remained steadfast for 4 years.

- All my digestive and gastro-intestinal troubles eased up and I could once again indulge in my previous so-called 'danger' foods e.g. bread and pasta. Also, my cravings for sweet and even salty foods diminished dramatically.

- Having experienced a little hormonal disruption and irregularity of my menses initially, regularity eventually set in after 4 months on MSM along with total freedom from pain and cramps. I no longer had any tenderness or throbbing pain emanating from my swollen ovary.

- Most importantly, approximately 70% of my melasma had cleared up after being on MSM for 6 months, despite these being predominantly the warmer spring and summer months of the year.

All these personal health improvements through MSM supplementation led me to believe that hormonal irregularities (caused by my swollen ovary) and Adrenal Exhaustion, possibly bordering on mild Adrenal Insufficiency (caused by prolonged emotional stress and years of prescription drug use), were predominantly to blame for the development of my melasma.

So, it was with great trepidation and anticipation of any potential negative criticism that my findings may incite from the dermatology or scientific professions, that I decided to write this book. By doing so, my sole and honourable intention is to continue to help as many other women as possible whose luck in improving their melasma is all tried out. This book is to be regarded as a self-help book and is for general understanding only, and any MSM therapy for melasma is to be undertaken entirely of your own free will*.

Remember, despite the fact that it is known to be a very safe nutrient with a low toxicological profile, always check with your GP, dermatologist or nurse before you embark on this treatment.

Good luck!

---

* see Disclaimer

6

MSM Sulphur

All our bodies are composed, primarily, of five basic elements: oxygen, hydrogen, nitrogen, carbon, and sulphur, and sulphur, being one of the most abundant and essential minerals in the body is, unbelievably, one of the least researched.

MSM is short for Methyl-Sulphonyl-Methane, a naturally occurring sulphur compound and stable, odourless dietary metabolite of DMSO (Dimethyl Sulphoxide). MSM possesses similar biomedical properties to DMSO, but with none of the unpleasant side effects. It is a vital compound found in the tissues and fluids of plants, animals, and humans and, along with its related compounds, makes up 85% of the sulphur in living organisms. MSM is also made naturally in the human body from the amino acids methionine, cysteine and taurine.

Sulphur is necessary for:

• The formation of collagen, keratin and elastin and for building disulphide bonds that hold together the body's physical structure and tissues thereby helping to maintain their flexibility and elasticity.

• Maintaining cell membrane permeability, allowing cells to absorb nutrients and expel waste properly.

• Playing a role in tissue healing and repair.

• The essential formation of antibodies.

• The energy production within body cells.

- The formation of detoxification enzymes and the production of glutathione, one of the most important antioxidants found in the body.

Overall, MSM is, therefore, a very important mineral for healthy hair, skin, and nails, organs, joints and blood vessels.

Dietary MSM is found in eggs, raw meats, seafood, some fresh vegetables and fruits and milk. Processing of these products, even moderate processing, destroys or greatly reduces actual MSM content. Therefore, the human body, generally speaking, will be sulphur deficient unless raw meat and fish and unwashed and uncooked vegetables are eaten on a daily basis. MSM levels in the body naturally decline with age, so a combination of deficiency and decline are reported to result in symptoms of fatigue, tissue and organ malfunction, and an increase in susceptibility to disease. To be effective therapeutically, MSM should be taken frequently, ideally, every day. Researchers have generally used daily dosages of between 250 mg and 2,000 mg, yet in severe cases of deficiency, much higher doses have been used, and in some cases, without any major side effects at all.

MSM appears to be very safe, non-toxic (it has toxicity levels close to that of drinking water), non-allergenic and does not interfere or interact with any other types of pharmaceutical medicines. It is suitable for vegetarians, is GM free and manufacturers state that are no known contra-indications. However, most importantly, always check with your GP before taking MSM Sulphur, especially if you are taking any other medication e.g. drugs for unstable blood pressure or epilepsy. Caution should be taken if you are on blood thinning medication or aspirin or if you suffer from kidney disorders of any kind.

See my Questions and Answers chapter for typical queries regarding MSM supplementation for melasma that arose during the experiment.

MSM: Is this the Clear Solution for Melasma?

Exactly *why* MSM is proving to be very successful therapeutically in its treatment of melasma is relatively unclear and, being no scientist, I am left with no option but to attribute the scientifically proven benefits of MSM to its ability to treat the underlying aforementioned potential causative factors related to the development of melasma. In short, MSM seems to be able to tackle the underlying problems that precipitate the onset of melasma in the first place, which in my opinion, are not just hormone-related as many dermatologists presume. The following facts about MSM are derived from scientifically proven studies:

• It elevates cortisol levels thereby relieving the symptoms of mild Adrenal Insufficiency.

• It is a natural hormone balancer.

• It is a tyrosinase inhibitor, but it seems to prevent secondary browning reactions only, and only over-active hyperpigmented macules are targeted with the tanning mechanism of the normal melanocytes remaining unaffected.

• It is a powerful antioxidant; it aids in the production of glutathione (GSH), taurine, and N-acetyl cysteine (NAC) and other detoxification enzymes.

• It maintains cell membrane permeability enabling the proper expulsion of all toxins from body cells thus allowing nutrients to enter for health and repair.

• It appears to normalise collagen formation.

• It cleanses and purifies the blood, organs and body cells and tissues by means of binding itself to toxic waste, metals and chemicals, all of which are then excreted via the kidneys.

• It coats or lines the intestines thus enabling the eradication of pathogens adhering to the intestinal lining and allowing repair wherever necessary. Proper assimilation of dietary nutrients (particularly the B-group vitamins) and toxic elimination improves providing overall support to the possibly overburdened liver and kidneys and improving general health in the process.

• It is a pH balancer, balancing the body pH from an unhealthy acidic to a much healthier alkaline pH. Illness and disease (e.g. Candida) of the skin and body are found to be more common in those with a more acidic pH.

• It helps the body to absorb and utilise all of the crucial B-group vitamins more efficiently.

Some of the above factors could enable the body's immune system to recover its former health, especially if it has suffered from the long-term use of prescription drugs.

Another additional related therapeutic benefit could include:

• An increase in serum sulphate.

All of these factors, and any other as yet uncovered beneficial properties MSM may possess, and how they could directly affect (from a more scientific standpoint) its impact on melasma, will no doubt be revealed if and when further studies are carried out.

8

Questions and Answers

Q. Is MSM sulphur the same as DMSO, or the sulpha drugs (sulphonamide drugs), sulphites or sulphides that I am allergic to?

A. No, do not get confused between the two. MSM is organic sulphur and a vital nutrient. MSM presents organic sulphur in a form that the body can readily assimilate. It is a dietary metabolite of DMSO, however, whilst they both possess similar biomedical properties, MSM does not produce the unpleasant side effects that can be observed with DMSO. Sulpha-based drugs do not occur naturally and are used for the same purposes as antibiotics. Many people are allergic to sulpha drugs; however, no similar reactions have ever been reported with MSM. A third type of sulphur, the yellow elemental sulphur from chemistry class, can also be toxic to some individuals.

Q. How and where is MSM available?

A. MSM is available in capsule, tablet, powder, and crystal form and can also be bought in a readily available topical cream form. It is found in health food stores or can be bought online via the Internet.

It is important to supplement with a very pure brand, preferably one that is 99-99.99 % pure and has a trademarked logo stamped on the bottle. These trademarked logos guarantee purity of the product and any brand with these trademarks will be the safest and most effective to supplement with, as they are less likely to have additional fillers or additives in them.

There are also newer and stronger MSM brands available containing maximum strength MSM, which are found to be very pure, twice as effective and therefore twice as economical to buy as the dose (compared to the dose guidelines from ordinary strength brands) can, theoretically, be halved. It is wise to introduce these stronger formulas a few months into your MSM program in order to allow the body to adjust to lower strength formulas first, thereby reducing the possibility of any negative side effects.

It was found, during my relatively small experiment, that the use of an excellent quality brand did seem to have a direct bearing on whether there was an observance in the clearing of macules or not, especially where guaranteed purity was concerned. There are many rogue companies cashing in on the MSM buzzword and caution should be taken regarding checking out the purity of the MSM product they are selling. Whilst collating data, it did not seem to matter which of the many pure and trademarked brands were used, as all were capable of inducing changes to the macules. Some girls even switched brands regularly which seemed to temporarily speed up the changes in a few of them and prevented the body from becoming too accustomed to one particular brand.

Maximum strength MSM formulas were introduced at a later stage, having only become available or known about approximately five months into my experiment. They were instrumental to the rate and speed of recovery in a few of those who were already observing results, and induced changes in some sufferers who had previously seen none or very few results whilst using other, normal strength yet good quality, trademarked brands.

Q. How should I take MSM?

A. MSM can be taken with or mixed into any flavoured beverage or plain water. The powder and crystals tend to dissolve better in higher-than-room temperatures. It should be taken with food. The smallest dose that gives you the most benefit is optimal. More isn't necessarily better, just more. It is best to find, and you will know when you have found it, the dose that works for you as an individual. The body will use only enough MSM to meet its full requirements and any excess will be excreted via the urinary system, thereby wasted, so there is no danger of overdosing, just the danger of spending more money than necessary to keep your supplies up. Because the body excretes excess MSM after a 12 hour period, it is best to spread the full daily dose throughout your day in order to keep levels up for as long as possible during your treatment.

The dose recommendations given below are a guide only, because we all have different body sizes, weights, health factors and needs. 2000 mg (2 g) tends to work for general maintenance and health. However, more will probably be required for treating melasma and any other health problems present in order to make sure that not just the overall general requirements of the body are met first and foremost. However, too much too soon can lead to some minor side effects such as those outlined in the next question below. The more your body needs, the more you will be able to tolerate. An increased dosage may be needed during times of stress or illness.

Under supervision of a GP, some people have even been known to take very high doses and not suffer any adverse side effects. Dosages, mechanisms of action, and rationales for use are still being discussed in the scientific arena, and the low toxicological profiles of this phenomenal sulphur compound, combined with its promising therapeutic effects, warrants continued human clinical trials. It is important to be aware that, as yet, the FDA has not approved of this supplement and no RDA has yet been evaluated or supplied.

Generally speaking, during my experiment we took the following when supplementing with standard strength MSM only:

- 1 X 1000 mg capsule/tablet or ¼ level teaspoon powder/crystals for 2 days with breakfast

- 2 X 1000 mg capsule/tablet or ½ level teaspoon powder/crystals for 2 days with breakfast

- 3 X 1000 mg capsule/tablet or 1 level teaspoon powder/crystals for 2 days with breakfast

- 4 X 1000 mg capsule/tablet or 1 slightly raised teaspoon powder/crystals for 2 days with breakfast

- 5 X 1000 mg capsule/tablet or 1 heaped teaspoon powder/crystals for 2 days with breakfast

On reaching 5000 mg or 1 heaped teaspoon a day, to supplement further still, the additional doses were taken with lunch and/or dinner in the same format as points 1-5 above, until an optimal dose was found. This varied with each individual but tended to be on average between 8,000 mg and 15,000 mg/day. This dose was maintained for many weeks. Some girls found that they were more comfortable increasing their dose at a much more steady rate than that outlined above and they may have taken a few months to reach their optimal dose. It is wise not to rush in order to allow the body to adjust properly. Occasionally, circumstances dictated that a much lower dose had to be taken, e.g. during sickness or travel or through sheer preference, but this did not hinder progress in any way.

During cases where stronger, more concentrated brands of MSM were taken, either the dosage guidelines provided on the bottle were followed closely or they were boosted to suit the individual's own personal choice or tolerance levels.

Q. Are there any negative side effects?

A. Yes, a few. However, it is important to be aware that these side effects are experienced by only a low percentage of people, and sometimes only one or more of the side effects occur and always to varying degrees with each individual. After these symptoms pass, an increased sense of wellbeing, good health (both physically and mentally), and elevated energy levels are experienced by most.

Side effects can include:

• Gastro-intestinal problems (mild diarrhoea) and minor cramping

• Transient headache

• Puffy skin, mild water retention

• Wind/gas

• Tiredness

• Increased thirst

• Minor skin eruptions/breakouts

• Sleep disturbances

• Menstrual upset

• In very rare cases a rash can occur

- You may notice a 'metalic' taste in your mouth initially, but this will subside after a few weeks

- You may have a mild flare up of viral/fungal infections, particularly if they are lying dormant or if you are prone to them, e.g. verrucas, athlete's foot, tinea, thrush or cold sores

All of these symptoms are commonly related to the detoxification process and will pass after a few days or weeks. Cutting back on the dose temporarily and thereafter increasing at a more controlled and steady rate should bring about relief. Increasing the intake of fresh filtered or mineral water can help. Reducing alcohol and caffeine intake helps to lessen the severity of headaches and taking MSM with food also tends to decrease the GI upset. Taking smaller individual doses of MSM and dividing them throughout the day with food, instead of taking a high dose all at once, may be preferable. Sleep disturbances are alleviated by not taking MSM in the late afternoon or evenings.

Q. Is it better to take the crystal/powder form, OR, tablet/capsule form of MSM?

A. Personally, I think crystals or powder, because, in my opinion, they are more bio-available to the body. They are also purer and less likely to contain synthetic fillers and binding agents. You can also add the crystals or powder to a base to make a great topical gel (see below for details). However, newer, maximum strength formulas are available in tablet or capsule form and contain no synthetic fillers or binders at all. They are a particularly perfect solution for those who dislike the bitter taste of the dissolved powder or crystal formulas and, being available in the quick and easy to swallow form, are ideal for those who lead busy lives or travel a lot.

Q. Can I apply it topically?

A. Yes. MSM creams are readily available in health stores. But to guarantee the highest percentage of MSM available along with purity and quality, make your own topical by using your MSM powder or crystals and blending them into a base of your choice. This could be your regular moisturiser, but pure non-sticky aloe vera gel is best, which in itself provides therapeutic benefits for all types of skin conditions.

Add 1 level teaspoon of MSM to every single fluid ounce of base. This will give you a 17%-strength topical (the highest possible percentage that is available without the mix turning gritty) to use on the patches daily after washing both morning and night. Stir it well until fully dissolved, leave for a few hours in order for the MSM to dissolve fully and shake well before each use. It is better absorbed if applied to a non-towel-dried (damp) face. Not everybody used a topical solution during my experiment, proving that oral supplementation of MSM provided the most benefit. Whether a topical was used or not, all women remarked on how amazingly soft their skin on the whole became and how any other skin problems subsided through its regular use.

Q. Should I take anything with MSM?

A. Many people believe that taking at least one part Vitamin C - in the better, less irritating to the gut form of Ester-C - to four parts MSM aids its effectiveness. As such, despite having no clinical evidence to support this, many of us did take Vitamin C with MSM during the trial. I highly recommend taking a good dose of B-group vitamins with MSM on a daily basis.

Q. Is MSM safe?

A. It has been shown to have 1/7 the toxicity of table salt, i.e. it's 7 times safer than table salt. MSM, during some scientific studies, has been shown to have no negative side effects at 1 g per kg body weight, equating to around 68 g per day for a person weighing 150 lbs. N.B. Do not take at the same time as blood thinning or blood pressure medication and aspirin, or if you have epilepsy or any kidney disorder without first consulting your GP or nurse.

Q. Is it safe to take with my other medications?

A. Apparently, after many years of research, it has not been shown to interfere with any prescription medications. Sometimes, the effects of MSM can lead to a decreased need for prescription medications and can often replace them in due course (e.g. allergy drugs), but, as always, consult with your GP before decreasing or discontinuing your medication. Remember that it is also important to see your GP if you are already on blood thinning medication or aspirin, if you suffer from kidney disorders of any kind or if you are taking drugs for unstable blood pressure or epilepsy.

Q. I'm pregnant. Can I still take MSM?

A. Always check with your GP or nurse for professional advice. However, avoiding MSM completely would probably be advised.

Q. Does it smell offensive or taste horrible?

A. No, a pure, good quality brand is odourless and colourless when immersed in water and dissolves instantly leaving no residue. It has a slightly bitter taste, which can be disguised in flavoured drinks if preferred. The bitter taste subsides over time and becomes less noticeable as the body adjusts and body pH is balanced out.

Q. How long, if at all, will it take for me to see the effects of MSM on my melasma?

A. That depends on a few factors. Some sufferers start seeing changes within 12 hours and recovery is rapid, many notice results after 3-7 days, however, a few won't see any changes even after many weeks/months. Recovery rate could be relative to how long you have had your melasma or the underlying causes. No treatment, natural or orthodox, is 100% effective. Although the MSM success rate is high when compared to the few or non-existing results gained in trials studying methods of treating dermal melasma, until further extensive clinical studies are undertaken to ascertain why some participants in my study have not responded to MSM, we may never know for sure what the reasons for failure are.

Q. Will it be safe to take MSM for a long time?

A. Extensive studies have shown no negative drawbacks to long-term supplementation of MSM. People who take it regularly tend to have fewer colds and viral infections, but there have been no studies carried out to corroborate these anecdotal findings. MSM is not necessarily a cure-all, but some people do find that the beneficial effects continue even after they stop taking it.

Q. Will my melasma come back if I stop taking MSM?

A. It is unknown, as yet, whether your melasma will return afterwards, though I would consider it unlikely, especially if prescription drugs are avoided in the future (see next question below). However, if it is necessary for you to continue taking drugs, and a clearing of the macules is observed whilst also supplementing with MSM, then it would probably be advisable to keep taking MSM. It is trial and error.

Q. I am certain that my prescription drugs caused my melasma, why?

A. I personally believe that there is a growing trend of the over-farming of land and over-processing of food giving rise to a decline in dietary sulphur levels. Combine this with increased drug taking since the 1960's, then we could ask the question: could both these factors be the reasons behind the rise in incidences of melasma in recent years, especially where cases *un*related to taking the birth control pill or other hormonal drugs are concerned (the most commonly thought causative factors by the medical profession)?

Whether constant levels of dietary sulphur are necessary for protection from the effects of prescription drugs and their impact on, for instance, the adrenal glands, the delicate endocrine system and/or immune system, or whether the drugs themselves have a direct impact on existing body levels of sulphur, is unclear. This may explain why many cases of melasma, for the first time in years, begin to recede during MSM supplementation because body levels of sulphur are restored to normal, the hormones are balanced out naturally, and the possibly overtaxed organs like the adrenal glands and drug-impaired immune system return to their former health. In short, MSM seems to be able to tackle the underlying problem that precipitated the onset of melasma in the first place. This is my personal theory, and I believe that it warrants more extensive, scientifically controlled study.

During the MSM experiment, the main causative factor was indeed found to be the very drugs that many of us had taken, both prescription and hormonal, and their impact on the body. Many of the drugs taken, e.g. allergy drugs, seemed to have directly affected the hormone levels and/or increased photosensitivity and their long term use had affected the immune system, giving rise to common illnesses e.g. Candida, Irritable Bowel Syndrome, Leaky Gut Syndrome, Epstein Barr Virus etc. It was observed that many of these illnesses also improved on supplementation with MSM.

It must be borne in mind, however, that some girls had not taken any form of drugs at all, so, naturally existing hormonal irregularities withstanding, could a deficiency in MSM Sulphur alone play a role?

Q. Despite knowing that it caused my melasma, I have to keep taking the pill/prescription drug, will MSM not work for me then?

A. During my experiment, 4 months in, two women had to keep taking the birth control pill, and one, a thyroid drug. All observed changes to varying degrees. Unfortunately, other girls realised that the drugs they had to stay on were hampering their progress. Everybody will experience different results. Regardless of whether you are taking drugs or not, it helps to remember that MSM doesn't, unfortunately, work for everyone.

Q. What, if anything, could I expect to see happening?

A. Your melasma patches or macules could start to get tiny fragments, cracks and holes etc. appearing in them, that will gradually combine to form larger patches revealing normal-coloured skin. Fading occurs either at the same time or at a later stage. Some women observe the cracks and holes phenomenon, some observe just overall lightening, and others experience both. Changes will be sporadic, and superficial, lighter macules could change before the more stubborn, dermal melasma does or vice versa. Dermal melasma seems to metamorphose into epidermal over time which could then, with a degree of caution, be successfully tackled with bleaching creams or lightening agents too if preferred. However, it is worth knowing that epidermal melasma responds to MSM supplementation just as well as and at a faster rate than dermal. All areas of the face responded during the experiment; cheeks, nose, chin, forehead and upper lip, with the latter two seemingly being the most stubborn areas to treat.

Progress can be rapid initially, and after a few weeks, plateaus to a more even and steady rate. You may experience occasional 'quiet' days where nothing happens for a while; this is normal and does not mean that progress has stopped. It could take many, many months, even a year or more, until the macules have disappeared altogether, so patience is paramount. The length of time could depend on your age, overall health, how long you have had melasma and how widespread it is. It will also help if you protect yourself from the sun during treatment. Many women, except for the lucky few who have recovered at a rapid rate, are realistic and realise that they are in this for the long haul and could expect to wait up to a year or more for full clearance of the macules.

It is advisable to take photographs before you start taking MSM, and take them regularly thereafter. This will help you to ascertain whether you are experiencing changes whilst taking MSM, or not. A few of us, during 'quiet' moments, had periods of doubt about what we were actually observing facially, but the photographs proved otherwise, especially when compared with those taken a few months later.

Q. I have abnormal pigmentation on my body only, but not my face. Could MSM help this as well?

A. Yes, it can do. During the experiment, a few women had pigmentation on the neck, shoulders, arms, trunk and legs. MSM faded and cleared their patches as well. Hence MSM pigmentation treatment does not appear to be exclusive to the face alone. Remember, MSM therapy is rating below 100% in its efficacy, so it will not necessarily work for everyone.

Q. Does MSM have a bleaching effect then?

A. No. During this ongoing MSM experiment, it appears to be clearing the melasma permanently and reverting the abnormal pigment back to normal, and more importantly, safely.

Q. If I go in the sun, will I undo all my progress?

A. Some participants in this trial have already 'tested' their progress by brazenly facing the sun and discovered that any abnormal pigment in the macules that had reverted back to normal tanned in exactly the same fashion as the rest of the surrounding unaffected skin. This provided hope that MSM does offer a permanent solution to clearing melasma over time. Any abnormal pigment that still remained darkened a little, with or without sun protection, but not as much as before commencing the MSM program. It is comforting to know that, during my experiment, it became apparent that MSM seemed to protect many of us from sun exposure and the macules did not darken as much (if at all) as they would have done if not supplementing with MSM on a regular basis.

Q. Will it revert the pigment or affect the tanning mechanism of my whole body?

A. No. MSM seems to target abnormal pigmentation, overactive melanocytes or the underlying causes of melasma only, and unlike the popular whitening pills found in Asia, it will not lighten skin over the whole body.

Q. I have hypopigmentation in the form of Vitiligo/Tinea Versicolor/as a result of extensive use of Hydroquinone. Could MSM help this as well?

A. It is possible. Derived from the experimental data collated over the first 6 months of this MSM experiment, it came to light that a few women suffered from hypopigmentation due to prolonged use of hydroquinone, two suffered from Tinea Versicolor on their bodies, and two had medically-diagnosed

Vitilgo. All of these women observed pigmentary changes and announced that the patches were starting to look normal-coloured again.

Q. MSM is working for me I am sure, but my patches seem to darken again before menstruation. Does this mean that it has stopped working?

A. No, not at all. Many of us noticed during the trial that, despite the fact that the patches had lightened and/or broken up with MSM, our patches darkened a little due to the rise in hormone levels before and during menstruation. The darkening seemed to be most obvious in the few days prior to the onset of menstruation. Once menstruation had passed, the macules returned to their original colour and continued to lighten or break up over the ensuing months. It does feel like a temporary setback, but do remember to bear in mind that MSM can take months to return your skin back to normal, so try not to get too despondent.

Incidentally, stress can also make the patches more apparent due to the fact that hormone levels can go a little awry if stress levels are too high. So try also supplementing with Vitamin B-complex or indulging in relaxing activities that can take your focus and attention away from your condition may help, e.g. taking up yoga.

Q. I am using a topical bleaching cream at the same time, is this wise?

A. Why not? Some women in my experiment preferred to rid themselves of the dark pigmentation and its negative social impact as quickly as possible. I, however, preferred not to in order to be fully satisfied that the MSM alone was reverting my pigment successfully, permanently and safely with no other factors or treatments involved which could instill false hope in me. I was also aware of the alarming, potential dangers of permanent hypopigmentation occurring from overuse of some of the bleaching creams available and/or their ability to worsen dermal melasma. It is a purely personal opinion.

Q. Why is MSM not working for me?

A. There seems to be different 'types' of melasma or hyperpigmentation medically diagnosed as such (colour, pattern or site) coupled with different causative factors. It is unclear exactly how and why, until extensive clinical studies are undertaken, MSM actually works for some sufferers, and not for others. Underlying, but more serious, health problems could be hindering results and these would need to be tackled first, because getting to the core of any other problem, especially if it precipitated the onset of melasma, could be the key to your recovery. It may be worth trying the following:

• Improve your diet and try to introduce more wholesome organic foods and fresh fruits and vegetables. Cut down on your daily intake of sugar and salt.

• Try also incorporating a good quality brand of B-group vitamins on a daily basis (focusing particularly on B3, B5, Folic Acid and B12) into your regimen.

• Try introducing other powerful antioxidants such as Coenzyme Q10, Vitamin E or Selenium in addition to MSM.

• Increase your water intake and make sure it is filtered or bottled. Reduce your caffeine and alcohol intake.

• Make sure you are taking the optimal dose of MSM for your body size, weight and health requirements.

• Stop taking where possible, but only with your GP's consent, any prescription drugs that could be responsible for causing hormone irregularities, thereby inducing photosensitivity.

• Reduce your possible exposure to chemicals, both environmental, e.g. pollution, and topical e.g. creams, makeup, toiletries and sprays etc that may also be inducing photosensitivity or contact allergies. Try to only use sunscreens that contain safer non-irritating ingredients (titanium dioxide and zinc oxide).

• Get your hormone levels checked out by an endocrinologist.

• See your GP about whether an underlying disorder, e.g. Addison's disease is present that could require specialist treatment first.

• Try switching to a purer and/or stronger brand of MSM.

• Indulge in relaxing activities, such as meditation, in order to reduce your stress levels. Assess your lifestyle; if you have a stressful job, try changing it. A B-group vitamin deficiency can result from continuous stress, not to mention the negative impact that stress can have on the adrenal glands!

• Be more patient! Some women took 3-4 months to observe any change at all during my experiment. Depending on the causes, the longer you have had melasma, the longer it could take to see results, so don't give up!

Q. Is there anything else I should know?

A. You will gain many other physical and emotional health benefits by taking MSM presenting themselves in many different forms, and they will be individual and unique to you and your current health situation. Only then will you be able to truly ascertain what has improved physiologically and conclude how it may have borne any relationship to how or why your melasma appeared in the first place.

9

Testimonials

All of the following testimonials (some provided on a periodic basis) were kindly given by just some of the women who took part in my experiment during the first 6-month period of the trial only. Some of these testimonials could mirror your own personal situation and will therefore prove to be both informative and helpful in your possible recovery with MSM. Once the information in this chapter has been digested, it must be *your* decision entirely as to whether or not you try out MSM therapy for tackling your melasma. It is highly advisable to discover your own personal regimen and regulate it accordingly to suit you and your personal needs if you do decide to go ahead.

Any 'before', 'during' and 'after' MSM treatment photographs that any of the women involved have bravely supplied or wish to supply in the future, will be displayed on the 'Testimonials' page of my website at **www.melasma.co.uk** only, and these will be updated and added to whenever possible. The photographs supplied show changes observed that are attributed to the use of MSM Sulphur for the treatment of melasma only, and no other therapies, e.g. topical bleaching creams, were used by the individual throughout the whole period. None of the photographs, which have been taken by the women themselves in the privacy of their own homes, have been airbrushed or altered in any way, shape or form. Any changes in lighting are purely incidental and not intended to mislead.

*****

Ms K, Fort Lauderdale, Florida US

I started out at 1,000 mg per day of MSM for a few days, and then went up 1,000 mg every few days until I got to 4,000 mg. Around the 3rd or 4th day my melasma looked like it had lightened up some. Then I started experiencing the same things as you, as far as the little white dots and lines are concerned - really weird looking stuff - but it was normal skin-colored! I started getting puffy mostly in my hands and feet, so I have now cut down to 2,000 mg per day, which seems to be working for me. Like you said it is going so slow, but if it's permanent, it's worth it! I've tried everything in the past but the minute you go off of it, the melasma all returns. I feel so much better not putting any chemicals on my face, and I can go outside without worrying about the spots getting dark. I'm convinced that if I'd never started using any of those bleaching creams and chemicals that my melasma would never have gotten so bad. I'm finally starting to feel normal again. So, thanks for all the advice and encouragement because it seems to be working for me!

*****

Yesterday I went to a baseball game, which was at 1pm, and it was a very sunny South Florida day. Our seats were in the beating down sun of course, which a couple of months ago would have made me panic! Well not only did I not panic, when I got home I washed my face and the existing spots did not get any darker at all! This was after 4 hours of primo sun exposure wearing just a baseball hat!

Ms LW

I have been on MSM for about 1 ½ weeks, I am starting to see results just as Ness described white spots and cracks where the melasma has been for years and they are the same color as my skin. I did not have many side affects and I feel great now, my body was detoxing a bit at first now I feel better than ever.

Ness, thank you so much - I wish I could have spent all the money on numerous consultations with the dermatologist on you. You are the best.

*****

I am having some very rapid results. Every morning I wake up I have new white spots and cracks where the melasma has been for years!

*****

I am so happy to report that my melasma is at least 90% gone. It has lightened and disappeared.

Ms D, UK

I have now been on MSM for 7 days and have been taking the powder form at breakfast, lunch and in the evening. I have also been applying it topically morning and night. I have now worked my way up to 6000 mg per day (with no side effects, drinking gallons of water!). Anyway at first I thought it was just wishful thinking but after a very close inspection I can now see about 7 or 8 white spots on my cheeks and this morning I discovered a complete patch missing! It is definitely not my imagination! It is only about the size of a 5 pence piece but nevertheless, it is there and I feel on cloud nine!!! My dark patches on my forehead and chin, which are very dark, have shown no results yet but my cheeks are definitely showing signs of improvement.

*****

My cheeks are definitely still fading in colour and also the patches are getting smaller. I had a very defined "mask" of brown pigment with about half an inch of white skin around the very edge of my face near my ears. Well now that white area is moving in and about 1½ inches of clear skin is now showing. So my patches are definitely shrinking! I know this for sure because I measured them!

I feel so much more confident and attractive than I have for years. My patches on my cheeks are still shrinking and as I reported the other day my very stubborn (hot chocolate) chin now has 3 patches in it! I have not had any 'cracks' to date, only white patches that slowly join up with other white patches.

I will repeat what I said to you in the early days of your discovery of MSM (Author: for the treatment of melasma) and that is that it has done more for me than any anti-depressant ever could. And for the first time in years I have got some confidence back. I will also say that I think I am about 30% clear around the edges of my "mask" and it is a good few shades lighter. I am not yet able to go without makeup but it will come.

I also wanted to say to you that apart from your determination in this crusade I for one think that you are very brave to have used yourself as a guinea pig in the first instance, I know lots of us have followed your lead but it still takes guts to try it first and then have the confidence to post it to all of us desperate women because lets face it that's what we all are. We have all been let down so often and spent thousands of pounds trying to cure ourselves only to find that our melasma just keeps coming back.

Ms LD, Sunshine State US

I started taking MSM on March 22nd 2002. I'm up to 6000 mg per day and 1000 mg Vitamin C. I take 3 capsules, (1000 mg each) in the morning with 500 mg of Vitamin C & 3 capsules in the evening with the other 500 mg of Vitamin C. Because I didn't have any side effects I upped my dose every two days. The recommended dose is 6000 mg per day. I drink water but not as much as I should.

When I started taking MSM I was not expecting results right away - I was prepared for a long haul; after all I've had this skin disease since 1981. However, like everyone who's posting results I have noticed the white spots. Also I've noticed that as a whole my face is starting to lighten, as if I were using a bleaching cream, which I'm not, that is wonderful! I had patches on my neck that looked like two thumbprints. They appeared out of nowhere about a year ago. I knew that it was the cursed melasma. While inspecting my face for changes I noticed that the two thumbprints are almost GONE! I had forgotten to check that area so the results were noticed right away.

*****

Now for the good news: I started MSM sometime in late March. It's definitely working but very SLOW. However, I didn't expect an overnight miracle after all I've had this condition for many years. As for me it doesn't matter how long it takes, something positive is happening. From what I can see it looks like it's working its way from bottom to top. Fragmentation is taking place on the chin and cheeks while it's lightening all over. I guess the forehead will be the last to go. Overall I'm happy with the results. Thank you Ness for your research and discovery (Author: of MSM's ability to treat melasma). Don't give up girls - patience is the key word!

*****

There's no doubt in my mind that MSM works. It does seem to stop but my theory is that our body gets used to it. In my case I changed brands, lowered/upped the dose depending on the amount I was taking or stopped taking it for a while and started all over again. That's what I did; I ran out and didn't get around to buying it for week or so. I purchased a new brand of MSM powder with Vitamin C. So far everything seems to be going great!

*****

One of the things I've notice, people expect an overnight relief...it's not going to happen! We need to be practical. Though some of the melasma seemed to appear overnight it's not going to go away just like that. I've been dealing with melasma since 1981, if you calculate correctly that's a lot of years! What started as a small patch turned into a horrible disfigurement to the entire face and neck! Yet, MSM seems to be working for me. Everyone that knows my condition and me has noticed the difference. My face is much lighter and the melasma is breaking up.

*****

Quick scenario: I am Latin/Italian decent, female, 56 years old. I'm overweight because of an accident, I was not when I developed melasma. Now I am able to workout again and the weight is coming off, thank goodness. I live in the Sunshine State. I wear sunscreen (without Parsol, it didn't agree with me). I even wear it before sitting by my computer. Yes, the monitor aggravated my melasma. Unless you're one of the lucky ones, I would wear sunscreen (your choice of brand), all the time. I apply the MSM powder and aloe mixture in the morning when I wash my face underneath the sunscreen. I do the same in the evening underneath any night cream I might wear. Ness, I am grateful for your diligence and determination. Personally I feel that you're onto something.

Ms J, Sacramento, California US:

I started taking the MSM about 10 days ago. I started with 2000 mg MSM per day with 1000 mg vitamin C and 500 mg calcium (just because I need calcium). 3rd day I increased to 3000 mg MSM and on the 5th day after no side effects, I increased to 4000 mg MSM per day then 2 days later (7th day) I increased to 5000 mg per day. Still no side effects and the 9th day I increased to 6000 mg per day. I'm still taking 1500 mg Vitamin C and 500 mg calcium per day. I mixed the MSM powder with aloe as suggested and have been applying it morning and night.

I noticed the light spots (and it may have been wishful thinking) around the 5th day. But last night I noticed the breaking up of the brown patches; it's faint and around the edges but it's definitely improving.

*****

I thought I would give an update on my progress...Last night after I washed my face I was doing my nightly inspection for progress and I thought my face was starting to break out. It looked like there were little spots all over my cheeks. Upon closer inspection, I realized it is little white spots in the middle of the brown pigmentation that is all over my cheeks. I believe that it's the MSM creating new skin cells that are normal!! I really do think this is working!!!!

*****

I have upped my dosage to 8000 mg per day. I was a little down last week not really seeing any results in the cheeks, just the forehead. Over the last few days, I have noticed the forehead is really fading as well as breaking up and the cheeks are indeed lightening. I am so amazed!! I can't wait to take my next dose!! Since taking the MSM I have noticed that the melasma does not get darker after a day in the sun, and although I am extremely faithful with the sunscreen, a day in the sun does not set me back in my improvement.

*****

My melasma seems to be lightening a lot. My forehead has lightened significantly. I'm still on 8000 mg a day and applying topically twice a day. The best benefit that I'm experiencing though is the fact it's not getting worse in the sun. I play golf once a week and although I wear a visor, in years past the melasma would get darker each time I was exposed to the sun no matter how much sunscreen I used. It's not worsening at all since taking the MSM. I feel like I have my life back!!!!!

*****

I have melasma with the seemingly common octopus markings on my forehead, the makeup line around the hairline and the melasma covers my lower cheeks on both sides and each side has a completely hyperpigmented spot from previous chemical peels. I first noticed melasma when I was taking the pill about 20 years ago.

I began taking MSM April 4th. I take a pure brand from the US, 1000 mg caplets and the crystal powder. I steadily increased my dosage every 2 days by 2000 mg until I am now taking 8000 to 9000 mg per day orally and putting the powder mixed with aloe vera gel on my face topically twice daily. I saw results around the 7th day. The melasma on my forehead started cracking and has lightened everywhere. The cheeks have a mottled effect. Since taking the MSM I have noticed that the melasma does not get darker after a day in the sun, and although I am extremely faithful with the sunscreen, a day in the sun does not set me back in my improvement.

I only experienced minor side effects in the beginning - a slight headache and nausea. I am a little more sensitive to a hangover after drinking (not nearly as bad now as when I first began taking the MSM). Positive side effects: skin is smooth and clear. I have a scar on my left palm that began itching after my 2nd week on the MSM. At first I couldn't figure it out, but the scar is almost gone now and the itching has stopped. Nails and hair seem healthier.

Ms O, Brooklyn US:

Something is definitely happening. The melasma continues to fade. This morning I woke up and another swathe was cut through a solid block, which ran from above my left eye to the area below the eye. I had two recent 'getaway moments' with gas but never linked it to MSM. Now imagine an etiquette teacher walking on a sidewalk and having a string of 'bullets' escape. I was as shocked as the woman walking behind me who made an immediate dash for the other side of the sidewalk. To say I was embarrassed is putting it mildly, but I had to laugh as I thought 'serves her right for tailgating'. Yesterday it was a burp that came totally out of the blue - again I was on the sidewalk. However, the man who was about to overtake me laughed so hard, that the two of us ended up laughing until we doubled over. It was a great moment that lightened my day.

Ms C, New Zealand:

I had been using a bleaching cream for some months to great success - however, I noticed that my spots would still brown in the sun and I still retained some telltale pigmentation on my face even after 12 weeks. I started using MSM 5 weeks ago and my melasma is all but gone now. When I think about the torture I went through with this skin disorder - I cannot believe how great my skin is now!

*****

Now for an update: I am still taking MSM - only 2 x 1000 mg capsules per day - more than that has side effects like aching, feeling like I am dehydrated and a weird kind of "spaced out feeling". All of these are pretty mild, however, they are recognizable and were enough to make me cut back to 2 tabs a day.

*****

Over the last 6 weeks (Author: Ms C was still using bleaching cream as well as MSM) the melasma on my lip remains practically totally cleared. I can confidently wear no make up and the lip area is not at all noticeable. You are probably sick of hearing this, however, you have been a god send to so many women and you are very kind for helping us deal with this awful condition - when so many doctors etc couldn't care less OR could not offer a solution.

Good on you!

Ms K, Illinois US:

I am 35 years old and have 2 children. I have taken many different kinds of BCPs since I was 17 years old. BCPs seemed to be the only thing that would regulate my monthlies and take away the excruciating cramps that I used to get when I was younger. I have always eaten reasonably well and I am 5'8" tall and weigh 123 pounds so I have always been on the lean side.

If I can remember back that far, I think my dreaded melasma appeared when I was about 6 months pregnant with my son. It came on very slowly but also in dark clumps all over my cheeks. I could not figure out what in the heck the dirty marks were that were appearing on my face. The OB doctor told me what they were and said that they would disappear shortly after giving birth. Well, doc, I'm still waiting! I tried every over-the-counter fade cream and every kind of lotion with AHAs and BHAs, etc. I never ever got a prescription for any type of fade cream either. I heard from my friends how irritating they were on there skin so I chickened out. I have also never had a prescription for acne.

I haven't been to a dermatologist, but I just know that my melasma is dermal. I ordered the MSM, and I think I started with about ½ level tsp and gradually increased the dosage after 3-day intervals. I did have the headaches and occasionally some body aches when I would increase the dosage. Now, I am up to 2½ tsp twice a day. I also take multivitamins, 500 mg Vitamin C for every 1 tsp of MSM, and also calcium. I just wish I had taken up-close pictures of my face when I first started the MSM. I had a dark brown silver dollar size patch on my right cheek that has really, almost miraculously, faded away. It's not gone yet, now it's the size of a pencil eraser with some splotching all around it and much, much lighter.

I still have the yucky mustache on the left side of my upper lip, and I also have relentless dark splotches on both sides of my forehead. The left side of my cheek is scattered with melasma, not a real solid patch like the other side was. The splotches on my forehead and my lip seem to be the areas that are the hardest to get rid of.

Overall, I would have to say that my melasma has faded/disintegrated approximately 50%. I still have a long way to go. The silver dollar size solid patch that was on my right cheek has faded by about 85%!

Ms D, Connecticut US:

I started MSM about 5 weeks ago. My bottle of MSM said that ½ teaspoon was 1700 mg. I am taking about 2 to 2 ½ tsp a day. I will be upping that amount to 3 tsp as soon as I stop at the health food store to buy a new bottle. I ran out this a.m. My problem has always been on my upper lip and chin. I too am noticing a lightening. I was afraid to up the dose too fast as per the other girls. I eat very healthily, never do drugs, don't take medicines unless prescribed by a doctor for infection and only drink wine occasionally. I am hoping that the MSM will continue to make a difference. I was hoping for a faster lightening but will be patient. Good things come to those who wait.

*****

I am using about 2½ tsp a morning of MSM in my juice. I must admit that lately I am feeling like I have hit a plateau. My upper lip problem has definitely not gotten any worse; it seems to be lighter than it has ever been for a June (sun) time frame. I have been using sunscreen on my face every day. I am not sure if I should up my dose of MSM to 3 or 3½ tsp per morning. I also agree that after being outside I do not see it get darker like it used to. I teach kindergarten and must go outside for recess every day. I am happy with the progress (if a bit slow) but the June level of my face is much better than in past years. Slow but steady progress is much better than getting darker and darker throughout the summer. I must admit, I still use a retinoid skin cream on my face, but I use it all over. You know, to prevent whatever wrinkles I can at my age.

Ms P, Minnesota US:

After doing some research, I found this site and started MSM and have been taking it for about 5 weeks. My melasma has lightened and I am not experiencing any side effects from the MSM.

I will see how the MSM continues to work. Good luck! I am glad to hear that I am not alone with this problem.

*****

I have been taking MSM for almost 7 weeks. I never had the guts to have a picture taken before, but I do believe it is lighter. Now my rosacea on my chin seems to show up more because my melasma has lightened! I am from Minnesota and all my ancestors are from northern Finland. Many of my relatives have rosacea but I seem to be the only one with melasma. I spent many of my teen years tanning without sunscreens, which may have something to do with it? I am 49 years old and have had melasma for years, possibly 15 or more. I've tried the bleaching creams without much success and so have given up on them. I spend quite a few hours gardening and biking every day and usually every summer my melasma would get worse, almost black in some spots, but so far not this summer. I am so thankful that I found this MSM and am having some success.

Ms K, Barbados:

I've had melasma for years and been thro' all the traditional treatments but with nothing to show but an empty purse! My dermatologist obviously has nothing more to offer and I am not ready to be doomed to a lifetime of searching for the right shade of foundation (because I've had no success there either!).

What a joy it was to find you all. So, to cut a long story short, I'm taking 6g MSM daily (3 capsules twice daily). I don't know how good a brand it is but it was all I could find at the time. I also take 1000 mg Vitamin C (one of those effervescent jobs). This is my 2-week anniversary and something is happening!!! Actually, after one week I was sure there was a change but I thought I'd give it a bit more time. Anyhow, it's as Ness describes so I won't go into details.

I've been taking MSM 3 to 4 weeks now and the effects are noticeable, and not just to me. Now, you all are the only ones that know what I'm doing - I didn't make any announcements after all the previous failures...

*****

I feel so much better these days - especially emotionally. The MSM has worked a lot better than anything else I've tried and it's been a heck of a lot less traumatic than some of the procedures I've subjected myself to. I live in Barbados, I love to be outdoors too, and even if my melasma doesn't clear completely the MSM seems to be stopping it getting any darker - it's doing a better job than factor 50 sunblock that's for sure!

Ms J, Washington State US:

I was waiting to report on my success, since I wanted to be sure it wasn't just my imagination or wishful thinking. But I am now getting obvious clear patches and an overall lightening effect. Even if MSM does not work for everyone (and please give it time, I'm sure it may even take years for some people to see an effect), this is your best hope for curing melasma; I can guarantee you will not find anything else out there!!!

Just be patient...

*****

I have had melasma on my forehead, cheeks and chin for about 13 years and have tried everything that my dermatologists have recommended, to no avail. I started MSM in April, and am now taking 8 grams of MSM crystals daily and Ester-C. I have noticed an overall lightening effect of about 25%, but the biggest improvement is on my forehead. My forehead now has a big clear chunk of normal pigment in the middle and the top and sides are fragmenting. I've also noticed that my skin is very soft and my two ugly little toenails are now growing in normal.

Ms L:

Here's news: my forehead blotches (dark, creeping, wretched things) have not budged. But my icky mustache has lightened! Is it usual for some spots to go before others do so?

As for microdermabrasion? NO, NO, NO! I underwent a series of six, at the "reduced" cost of 100 bucks a pop (!) and I was left with three brown scars where the sandblasting went too deep (as I mentioned, I hyperpigment when I scar), and my melasma? FULLY INTACT! It was a costly lesson indeed. Hopes still high!

Ms D, Tampa Bay, Florida US:

I am the Florida girl who was diagnosed with melasma on my arms, shoulders, and neck. I have been taking MSM for over 3 weeks now. I still plan to increase my dosage to achieve quicker results. I started slow, but plan to get up to 6000 mg. I have been taking 2000 mg of MSM, applying MSM powder and aloe vera gel mixture to my skin, and drinking lots of water. I am also on a detox/cleanse program because I have had a past of problems with digestion and elimination. I am seeing my melasma fragment, crack, dot and also begin to fade. I am so happy!!

Thank you Ness for educating me about MSM. You have helped many people.

*****

I am so happy with my MSM results. I will keep you posted on further results. I also want to report that my melasma is not getting any darker from the sun. My boyfriend, family, and friends have noticed the difference in my skin. It is great when others notice.

*****

My melasma continues to fade. Every day I take MSM and vitamin C plus an application of MSM and aloe vera gel on my skin at least once a day.

Ms D, Chicago US:

I have held off reporting on my success with MSM. I have used it approximately for 7 weeks and was not sure I was getting results, but now I do believe I see the 'scratches' Ness is talking about. I have upped my dosage to 10,000 mg in the last week. My melasma has never been solid patches and has always been mottled so the progress is harder to spot. I really think all of these harsh chemicals used in treating melasma cause more harm than good. Hope some of you out there who are hesitant to use MSM change your mind.

Ms M:

I am a new one starting the MSM, and I too have a thyroid disorder, for which I am taking a particular drug. I have hypothyroidism, and am currently taking 7000 mg of MSM. I am taking a trademarked brand, and am starting to see results. I believe it is an answer to prayer, and I thank Ness's willingness to share this with all of us. I will post more, but I just wanted to let everyone know that I am seeing results. My melasma is starting to break up and it is indeed easier to blend with my makeup. Hang in there!

Ms E:

Ness, I recently started taking MSM. I jumped onto the bandwagon on Wednesday night. As most of you know, I have had melasma for about 6 to 7 years, and have tried everything to get rid of it. I am absolutely THRILLED to report that after only 4 days of MSM I see results. My moustache is beginning to fade, and I keep going to the mirror to check it out throughout the day. I haven't seen the cracks that Ness has referred to, but I have noticed an overall lightening of the entire thing, especially on one side of the moustache. The other side, which has always been a little darker than the other is fading, and there are two very faded spaces in that part of the melasma. I feel like I have a new face, and it feels wonderful.

I also have two patches that are about the size of nickels on my cheeks. They were light to begin with, and they are also lighter, although the difference in the moustache has been the most remarkable difference so far. It is amazing to me to think that after years of struggling with melasma, in a matter of just a few days, I am returning to the person I used to be with the confidence I had years ago. The side effects I have experienced have been mild but noticeable. I have had the "transient headache" and I have been thirsty. The benefits far outweigh the side effects, so I am going to continue with MSM.

*****

I have been taking MSM for almost 7 weeks. I am taking the trademarked powder form of MSM orally. I started at 2,000 mg per day and gradually worked up to 4,000 mg per day, which is the recommended dose on the jar. I began to see results of lightening in the dreaded moustache after 5 days. It seems as though progress was very fast at first, then slowed down. That trend continues, yet it seems just when I think the pigment has not lightened in a while, soon afterward (within days) I will notice that it does in fact look lighter. The only real set back I experienced was the week before my period. It looked darker that week, but lightened up again the next week.

From the time I began MSM to now, on a scale of 1 to 10 with 1 being light and 10 being dark, I started out as a 10 and the melasma is now at 5. I have a two-part moustache that is divided by a clear spot in the middle. The right side is now lighter than the left for some reason. I also have melasma in two spots on each cheek which I have not noticed much change in. I really don't care so much about these spots; rather, it is the upper lip curse that I am closely following. The progress is thrilling. I am praying that everyone will see positive results.

*****

I am 3 months pregnant now, and I am not taking any MSM. All I wear is sunscreen. I was concerned before I got pregnant that I might have a darkening of the melasma if I were to conceive. I'm pleased to report that the melasma is no darker now than it was before I got pregnant. I believe that taking MSM before getting pregnant helped to lighten the melasma and keep it light.

Ms D:

I don't want to jump the gun here but I may be seeing some differences in my melasma. My mustache looks different - kind of splotchy. I have been on the MSM 6g a day for about a week or so. If it is actually changing than I am going to be so happy…

*****

I have melasma on my upper lip and a tiny bit on my cheekbones. It looks like two splotches on either side of my lip like a mustache. I have had it for almost three years now and I can still remember the day that I first noticed it. I started MSM almost three weeks ago. I started with a trademarked brand of MSM (capsules) at 2g a day until I got another trademarked brand (powder) in the mail and then I upped my dosage steadily. Now I am on 8g per day. I really think I saw some changes after about 5 days on the 6g dose. I saw fragmenting, sort of like little dots. Actually, it seems to be slowing down a little over the past week so I think I might change brands again and up the dosage. I have been using oral MSM only in the mornings and topical at night. I have had no side effects except for some insomnia so I only take the MSM in the morning. I am very prone to insomnia so I may have just been paranoid, and it may not have been caused by the MSM at all. Now I am symptom-free (knock on wood).

Ms M, Florida US:

Well Ness, I think I may see a tiny little break up of the melasma on my chin. I may have a real heart attack if this lightens up and eventually disappears.

*****

I am also happy to report that the melasmic activity I have did not change after a 5-hour day at the beach in South Florida. I applied my sunscreen, and of course makeup, wore my hat for a while and finally said screw it all, just to see if it would come back. I went swimming in the ocean, lay on the chair and as soon as I came home, practically ran to the mirror to stare at my face. As of this morning if there is anything I have noticed, it is that the hot chocolate chin seems to be more speckled looking instead of a large patch.

To be honest I am hoping to rid my face of the hairless mustache, but feel very encouraged now that my beach day has not made matters worse.

*****

I have melasma on my chin, (the chocolate ice cream effect) the mustache and several areas of old scars that heal very dark from a dog bite and assorted other mishaps. I also have hypopigmentation along my cheeks creating white blotches where there used to be normal skin, this is from a chemical peel and laser treatments which I used to try to cure me of my melasma.

I began taking a trademarked brand of MSM about 2 ½ weeks ago. I started out on 500 mg a day and am now up to 6000 mg per day, taking 3000 mg in the morning and 3000 mg in the evening. I take 500 mg of Ester-C along with the MSM. I have only had one minor side effect, which is the transient headache, but it does seem to be relieved by drinking more water. I also use an MSM cream, bought in the health food store.

I began to see results after 8 or 9 days, whilst taking about 4000 mg of MSM. I have noticed that the edges around the chin don't seem to be so pronounced and defined. The cracks and dots that have appeared within the chin area have made the melasma look more mottled. I have also seen a dramatic improvement regarding sun exposure; I live in Florida where sun is a constant factor. Well I am happy to report that I have now spent the last 3 days sitting on the beach and have had no darkening of the melasma. Also the scars that I have from the dog bite have not darkened despite the sun bathing at the beach, the scars from that are right on my shin bone.

Plan for the future: once this trademarked brand of MSM is gone, I will buy a different trademarked brand, or may even mix the 2 brands together, using 3000 mg of one in the mornings and 3000 mg of the other in the evenings. I plan to increase the dose I am on by about 500 mg a week.

Thanks again Ness for all your hard work and devotion!!

*****

Well Ness I have got to tell you, its definitely working for me. It is not so much as I have a few areas that have the 'dots and slashes' but it is getting lighter every day. Not only is it lighter, but also my skin seems much smoother, especially where the scars are from the chemical peel. For all of you who are skeptical, don't give up too soon. It is obvious that each individual will progress at his or her own pace and therefore results will vary. I am currently into my 4th week on MSM having gone from 1000 mg to my current dose of 7000 mg a day along with Vitamin C. As far as I can tell the mustache (the one thing I hate the most) is lighter by about 5 shades. This is the one area I want GONE!

Ms BV, US:

You are wonderful. Thanks for doing this for all of us. So far I am doing fine. I will go to 5000 mg next week. I took some pictures and compared them with last month's pictures, I think I see my melasma is lighter... but I will take the pictures again tomorrow for sure.

*****

MSM really WORKS!!!! Yeah!!!!!

Ms C:

I have been silent until now - until I was convinced 'something' was really happening. I had been on the birth control pill for a number of years with no problems. I have always been a very outdoorsy person, in the sun all the time again without problems. Then, when I was trying to get a little color so I would look good for my wedding I developed this wonderful condition. Cruel irony huh?? My husband surprised me with a honeymoon in Jamaica. My first trip to sun and sand and I couldn't even relax and enjoy it! Anyway I have tried all the same creams that most others have tried and the only thing that keeps this somewhat under control is living like a vampire, avoiding all the activities I so enjoy and avoiding the outdoors at all costs.

I read Ness's posting about MSM a few months back. Well I decided to go for it. I ordered some MSM off the Internet. I was so impatient that I couldn't wait and went to my local pharmacy and purchased 1000 mg tablets. It is a trademarked brand of MSM. Well I worked my way up to the 5000 mg per day and thought the spots were fading and maybe feathering around the edges a little. I kept upping the dosage to 8000 mg and then I ran out of the product I purchased at the pharmacy so I began using what I got from the Internet for about two weeks. I have to say that the progress seemed to stop. I was so disappointed. I thought I had been imagining it all.

Then I decided to go back to the pharmacy and get more from them. I am now up to 10,000 mg and thrilled to see huge cracks in the most offending part of my moustache. So brand does matter. That is why I am finally posting my results. When I began 8 weeks ago, I decided I would admit that I was having results if and only if the moustache began to go. My skin also looks and feels better than it has done for years. My acne is much better and my skin in general is not as oily.

One other interesting effect is that since going off the pill two years ago I would always be able to tell exactly when I was ovulating. Very sharp pains around my left ovary for about 12 hours, always 14 days before my period. This has disappeared. I've been through 2 cycles without a hint of it. I have always been very regular and that hasn't changed. But the pain (which I didn't have when I was younger) told me my hormones were somehow different. I have to believe that the MSM is getting everything back to normal. I have to thank Ness from the bottom of my heart. Like others, people have noticed a different attitude. I don't hesitate to look people in the eye now. Before I would look away to hide my face.

Ness, you have given me the hope that I can have my life back. Maybe this summer I won't feel like a rat scuttling along the sides of buildings, or frantically searching for shade. Maybe a hat won't have to be a permanent fixture on my head any more. As for the side effects, the only thing I really noticed was the headache each time I upped the dosage. That went away after a few days.

Good luck to everyone who is on the MSM. I'm sorry it took me so long to post results, but I had to be sure my eyes weren't playing tricks on me. I can hardly wait until someone posts that it is completely cleared. What a great day for us all. And thank you Ness for being a light in the darkness and despair for all of us. We are all in your debt.

*****

It has been 4 ½ months now, now up to about 12 000mg per day - overall fading and some total breakup.

Ms R, US:

Ness's results with the MSM convinced me to purchase a bottle that very same day. I have melasma that started 7 years ago on my upper lip, progressed to the upper part of my forehead, then last year my entire chin (looks like I dipped my chin in chocolate ice cream!) under both eyes, so I look like I'm wearing a mask, and lastly over the middle of my forehead with tentacles over both eyebrows – the 'octopus'. Pretty well 90% of my face is covered. My melasma is the result of birth control pills and excessive sun.

I started taking MSM on 4/18/02. I could only find a non-trademarked brand at the local health food store but on 4/28/02 I started taking a trademarked brand and lotion. I'm taking the capsules, 3 at breakfast and 3 at lunch for a total of 6 grams a day. I slather the lotion on three times a day. I didn't notice any results until last night. It looks like my forehead patch has cracks and is fragmenting. This morning I closely examined my cheeks and I can see white spots! I really feel like switching to the trademarked pure brand of MSM made a difference in my progress. I haven't experienced any side effects besides some excess air and feeling nausea in the morning after taking the pills. Some good side effects are that my skin is very soft, not oily, my hair seems softer too and shiny, my nails are growing faster and I have more energy.

I would like to thank Ness for finding and researching MSM (Author: for the treatment of melasma), I thought I would have to live with melasma the rest of my life and now I have hope. I dream of the day I can go makeup free and let my bangs grow out! I'm going to Florida in June and hope I will be able to stay in the sun without my pigmented areas getting darker. I will keep everyone updated on my progress.

*****

As for an update on my progress - this morning I noticed three spots on my chin, which is where my melasma is the darkest. I also noticed that one of my tentacles has broken away from the large patch on my forehead. Proof that it is patch is indeed shrinking. My cheeks seem to have more spots too. I'm hoping at this rate in a few days that the patches on my cheeks will look more like freckles.

*****

My progress report is as follows: I've been on the "pure" MSM for almost 2 weeks; I have upped my dose to 8 g a day. I'm having very good results; my second tentacle has broken away from the patch on my forehead. The patch on my forehead is shrinking and one corner on my forehead is nice healthy skin, however the patch now has such a bizarre shape, almost like a stair step effect.

I'm very pleased with the progress on my cheeks. When I started out the melasma on my cheeks looked like a mask. Now there are clear spots of skin within the patch, and the patches have really shrunk dramatically. My chin also has the clear spots. I haven't really experienced any detox side effects. My energy level is incredible.

Best of luck to all!

*****

The MSM I take has Methyl-sulfonyl-methane 99% and water 0.1% and nothing else in it. I had results after just a few days of taking it. I didn't start taking Vitamin C with it until last week, and I don't think my brand of Vitamin C is the Ester-C type; it's the cheap stuff. I hate to hear that not everyone is seeing results with the MSM it has been the only thing that I have had results with after 7 years of melasma. I feel that it's a 'cure' for me, and I also like that it is safe, cheap and healthy. My skin has never been so soft and smooth and I actually have nice nails.

For all newcomers, I would highly recommend trying it and for those it's not working for, evidently it doesn't work the same for everyone or it just takes longer.

I wish I had taken a photo before I started with the MSM treatment so everyone could see the difference now after almost a month. The melasma on my cheeks has shrunk almost by 50% but the forehead and chin are going much slower.

Ms L:

Well I have been on MSM for 5 days now and I must say to Ness: "As far as I am concerned you have earned yourself a pair of wings!" I first noticed my melanoma (on upper lip mostly) but I do have little freckle spots on cheeks and forehead going on now for 2 years. Anyway I wanted to be sure before I made my posting that I was not just seeing what I wanted so badly to the changes that are now starting to take place. I have always had dry skin and experienced a general tightness to it. After just one day of taking MSM the tightness is gone! My skin and eyes have more brightness to them and the freckle spots on my cheeks and forehead are starting to fade a bit. I also have noticed my upper lip is lighter than the usual shade!!!! My makeup is now starting to conceal and blend nicely.

Ms R, Sweden:

Well I also have been on MSM (8000 mg for a week) and haven't noticed too much improvement except that the melasma doesn't get worse in the sun! That's great news for those who want to stay on the pill. I think though if I am going to clear myself of this I will probably have to stop the pill. But I am still going to give it another month on birth control. But I LOVE MSM, no spring allergies and nice hair and nails, thanks Ness!

*****

I am one of those who are still on the pill and have taken MSM for almost a month now (4000 mg twice a day of a trademarked brand) so I thought I would give an update. I just got back from Spain tonight and have good news my melasma didn't get worse! I even lay on the beach for three days wearing an SPF 15 (stupid but I needed to know) and was able to get a tan. Unfortunately I don't see much of a change in the spots I already have, but I feel that has to do with the pill I am on. It is great though that I can finally enjoy the sun again without being scared of the outcome. I found by being in a warm climate that my headaches increased and I was thirstier. Even though I haven't seen so much of a breaking in my spots I will definitely stay on MSM because I, for the first time, don't suffer from my spring allergies, sleep better, my skin is smooth and I can eat chocolate again (my food allergy)!

Ms O, Israel:

I want to update you on my progress. I started taking MSM 12 days ago and to be honest, I didn't expect much...BUT it worked!!! I am on the birth control pill, I take antibiotics for prevention of cystitis, pluck my moustache and I live in Israel, which is sunny 99% of the time and I have had this melasma for 6 years ('moustache' and forehead dots).

Well - the right side of my 'moustache' became much lighter - first a light dot and then a bigger area, almost half of the right area! Those changes started only after a week, when my dose was 4000 mg. I stayed on that dose for a while and yesterday, in my 11th day, upped it to 5000 mg. Last and important thing: I want to thank Ness from the bottom of my heart. Not only that she found this amazing thing (Author: for the treatment of melasma), but for being there - answering, supporting, encouraging, caring and much more!!! It really changed my life and gave me a hope to start living normally!!!

*****

I also saw results after 6 days and now after 2 weeks, the right side of my moustache looks much lighter. I am still scared to check what will happen if I go to the beach, but I will soon...

Ms T:

I'm currently into week 4 of MSM - up to 10,000 mg per day with 1500 mg Ester-C (I just added the Ester-C – I hope this speeds up the process!) I have actually seen slight lightening of the 'octopus', but sometimes think it's just my imagination, but I will keep fighting it!! I do have a definite 'white spot' on my nose that used to be brown, so I'm hopeful that this is the 'cure' I've been waiting for!

*****

I came across this MSM phenomenon, so have decided to try a cheaper, more natural approach!! I'd like to say the results are incredible, but I'm not quite there...YET!!

Ms JR:

I am a 30-year-old female who developed melasma 3 years ago when I switched to a birth control pill that was suppose to be "good for the skin". Before that, I'd been on the BCP for 10 years with no adverse side effects. I developed a brown patch on my forehead, left cheek, and on my upper lip. I was prescribed a retinoid treatment with 4% hydroquinone. All it did was lighten the melasma. I could still see it even though friends said they couldn't notice. I tried a bleaching cream, no change, dermabrasion, some more lightening, but still the melasma was present. I stopped taking the birth control pill altogether.

After reading your message on MSM, I purchased 100% MSM powder, a trademarked brand, aloe vera gel to make the topical cream, and Vitamin C. I noticed white spots the very next morning!!!! After about a month, every dark area of melasma has been broken up with white patches!!! My cheek is about 95% gone, chin 50% gone, and forehead 50% gone. All areas are very light. I take about 10,000 mg a day and am working up to 12,000 mg a day. I have had only a slight headache in the beginning, which is entirely gone now. My diet is 'average' and I am a weekend drinker (dinners, clubs, parties, etc). My water intake hasn't changed, but that is all I consume during the day, save for a cup of coffee in the morning. I plan on taking MSM until every dark patch is gone!

Ms R, Michigan US:

I too am a new user of MSM. It is now three weeks. The info on detox symptoms scared me, so I started three weeks ago with ½ of a 1,000mg tablet and 500 mg of Ester-C. The second week I increased to 1 full tablet and same Ester-C. Now, I am in my third week (started June 3), on 2 tablets, which I take in the morning with the same amount of Ester-C.

• Results 1 - Holes in my melasma (cheek) that have increased every day! Saw results within 3-4 days. Overall lightening of the melasma - although it is still very noticeable.

• Results 2 - Lightened scar tissue on old surgery marks and a very dark scar on my leg. Some of the scar has turned white - the other parts have lightened. I expect the scar to be gone totally within a few weeks.

• Results 3 - I have a vaginal yeast infection. It has not gone away. However, the odor is very substantially reduced and the discharge is less.

• Results 4 - I used to go home after work (10 - 12 hours) exhausted and depressed. Now I am tired, but I do not fall into any depression-like behaviors, i.e. endless solitaire, sleeping, watching boring TV shows, worrying, feeling hopeless. I wake up with energy and enthusiasm and it lasts for most of the day.

• Results 5 - The first day I did not sleep for the entire night! I went to work very tired, but sleep did not overcome me until about 11:00 am at which I took a 10-minute nap and then moved on for the rest of the day. Insomnia for me has been frequent (depression) and I really worried about this effect of MSM. That is why I only take it in the morning. I'm afraid to split it into two dosages.

Overall, I am very pleased. I look forward to eliminating the melasma entirely and am prepared to go the whole year and longer to see it GONE FOREVER!

*****

I have been using MSM for two months now. Because I am a chicken to take anything - I don't even take tylenol or aspirins or vitamins, I was very leery of taking too much MSM for fear of reactions. So I took it very, very slowly. Started with 500 mg first week and then every week thereafter added another tablet of 1,000 mg. I am taking 1 g torpedoes and 1,000 mg of Ester-C. Today, I am up to 9 g of MSM a day – divided between the morning and afternoon.

I am very pleased with the results that I noticed within the first few days, i.e. small holes appearing within the melasma. I have two patches on each cheek that run down all the way to just above my jawline. The melasma on my left cheek (the darkest and largest) was in the shape of the map of South America. After 3 months, the Amazon River has increased in size, so that it looks like a waterfall down the entire map. Chile looks like it has fallen into the Pacific Ocean, pieces of Northern Brazil in the Atlantic and Argentina has lost its Cape.

The right cheek was the first to succumb (this was always the lightest and smallest side perhaps because it's the passenger side). The melasma is receding from the inside to the outside. Overall, the entire melasma on both sides have lightened by about 50%. It actually looks like the results of one or two light peels. I do not use any bleaching agents and I still try to walk out without any sunscreen. It's still very noticeable but I am thrilled. I am not afraid to go out without make-up if I have to, because the color is so much less intense.

The other benefits in health and attitude and skin are amazing. My hair is softer, skin is smoother, I have nails like iron and my scars are filled in and almost invisible, now. I still have a problem getting enough water now that I am back at work, and I notice that without it, I get bloating and headaches. I will increase to about 12 g. Then I plan to go onto high strength MSM and start my regime as if I am almost right back at the beginning again.

Ms A:

I have been taking the MSM (1000 milligrams) once a day since the time we last spoke. However, I have not taken it every single day. In addition to that I have had a micro-peel and have been using a bleaching cream also at the same time. As you can tell, I am determined to get rid of this plague! My melasma consists of two patches on both of my cheeks. The center of these patches has completely disappeared and in its entirety is much lighter.

The problem as you can guess is that I do not know which treatment caused these results if not in part all of them as a whole. If I had to guess, the bleaching cream did not do much since I had no significant benefits from prior use with it. The micro-peel I feel helped a lot and just as important as that I feel was the MSM combined with other vitamins like A, and E and eating healthy too!

Ms T, Queensland Australia:

I have had melasma for 1.5 years across my cheeks, side of nose, moustache, mildly dotted on my forehead. No idea why. I have taken no drugs, hormones, nothing only painkillers and anti-inflammation drugs. No BCPs or hormone or skin drugs. I started taking one trademarked brand, now I am another trademarked brand. And have been taking it for 2 months plus. I started noticing results after 2 weeks, whilst taking 4 heaped teaspoons a day. I am definitely about 6 shades lighter, can't see it at all in some lighting. It may be getting smaller around edges, but it's too light to see if it's breaking up. I have never tried any other treatments, this is the first thing I did after I found out what it was.

Ms S:

I would like to tell you that, although my melasma is not 100% cleared, I am definitely 90% clear. My hair is thicker and my eyebrows are thicker. I went back to 3 capsules in the morning and 3 capsules in the evening since 5-27-02 to give my body a break and it is still working for me. But one thing I know for sure is that MSM has become my lifetime supplement.

Take care and god bless you, just always remember Ness, I will never forget you because no doctor, nobody had given me hope for this melasma and as I have said, I do not feel so lonely anymore. Like you Ness, I cried so hard after two doctors told me that I must learn to live with my melasma because they can't do anything about it. But now that we have MSM, what more can I say except I am getting good results!

Ms LB:

First of all, I want to thank you so much for all the valuable information on MSM. This is the best research material I have ever come across on this subject and I truly appreciate all your hard work and dedication.

I have been working on finding a solution for my melasma for over 10 years. I've tried topical medications that initially improved the situation and then ended up making it worse. MSM is the first remedy I've tried that seems to be working. The progress is very gradual, but I am looking at a long-term solution so I'm willing to be patient. I initially started with the MSM capsules and then switched to the powder at the beginning of April. In my opinion, the capsules were worthless and the powder has brought about some results. I am currently taking about 6-8,000 mgs per day.

I am very confident that MSM will be the cure to this condition that has made me miserable for years.

Ms M, California US:

I'm 52 and have suffered with this for at least 20 years. I have dermal melasma REALLY BAD. Worse than I even realized until I started examining my naked face each day. I emphasize DERMAL because it's irritating to me when skincare specialists say that it can be cured easily with this or that cream or potion. It's important that people know that DERMAL is not easily cured.

For the past five years, I have had raccoon eyes with dark skin all around, spots appearing all the time on my face, an irritating rash on my neck that I now realize is melasma, and spots appearing on my legs (I have noticed on older relatives that they get a dark skin covering over their shins. Doctors always just tell them that it's because of poor circulation. Maybe, but it makes perfect sense to me that the cells are old and tired and that it's melasma).

Twenty years ago the only product was hydroquinone, so that's what I used on and off for at least 15 years. It would fade, come back, fade again, and reappear in other areas. For the past five years I have been trying every natural product that I could find, all types of bleaching creams, AHAs, etc (there were times when I would wake up with my face totally swollen from all the chemicals I was using). I have also at various times given up caffeine, cola, chocolate, carbohydrates, etc.

I went for two evaluations at the dermatologist, both suggesting I try expensive peels, dermabrasion, or laser therapy. It was something I was constantly saving for - but something more important would come up and the money would be spent. So I would start saving again. I now realize that it was a GOOD THING that I didn't have those procedures - surely it would have made my condition worse (not to mention wasting money that I didn't have)? They would also say that I must be in the sun too much and not using sunscreen. I don't like the sun. I've never spent much time in the sun. Even then, I felt like a failure. I must be doing SOMETHING wrong. But I couldn't figure out what it was.

I have probably spent $1000 in the last 3 years trying to find the answer. I always believed that it was a hormone problem that caused my condition - but that was just part of it (for the past year have been dealing with menopausal symptoms that have left me exhausted, and constantly bleeding – that is now under control with wild yam). I was now ready to tackle the melasma. I discovered all this talk about MSM. I did some research, read all about it and decided to give it a try. That was 10 days ago, Ness and it is TOTALLY working for me. I realize that it's going to take me at least a year to have significant improvement - but I am in this for the long haul. Especially since the benefits are so numerous. I must have been totally toxic and full of poisons. I live in San Jose, California, Silicon Valley, and the pollution and environmental toxins are probably everywhere I turn.

So far, my skin is noticeably clearing and fading. I see white patches appearing under my eyebrows and fading on my cheeks. The rash on my neck has stopped itching and is soft and smooth. My rough, bumpy elbows are soft. The stretch marks on my hips and thighs and breasts are fading. The heels of my feet even are smoother and any moisturizer seems to absorb easier and work better. I am taking a 500 mg pill every 4 hours. I don't really mega-dose on anything - I just like it nice and steady.

Thank you a million times. I now feel that I have a future without stares and strange looks. Nobody would ever say anything, but I could see his or her expression, i.e. "What is that on her face?" I feel more self-confident and have even started losing those extra 15 pounds that I've been working on for years. Melasma is not life threatening, but it does affect your self-esteem and quality of life.

*****

A quick update on my progress: I've been on MSM for about 2 weeks now:

• Noticeable overall clearing.

• My skin feels really soft.

• Eyebrow area starting to show color variation - like it's dissolving before my eyes.

• Big fingerprint-size glob below one eye - this one had little bumps on it - skin starting to heal and lighten.

• Donut-shape spot on my cheek - about the size of a fingerprint - inside starting to whiten and outside getting uneven edges.

• Neck area clearing up.

It's funny that I have it all over, but no mustache. Go figure! I know I'm going to reach a plateau soon. I'm just so happy with the progress so far. I also realize that it doesn't work like this for everyone. But the point is that we're heading in the right direction. Don't give up the fight.

PS: Thanks Ness.

Ms K, US

I, believe it or not, have both melasma *and* vitiligo. How I wish I could just cut and paste my skin and put the dark spots where I have no pigment at all. The vitiligo is confined mainly to my extremities, however, I do have it on my eye lids. The melasma is on my forehead and cheeks. Anyway, I started MSM two weeks ago; I'm up to 7000mgs.and may have minimal results (Author: with the melasma), it's hard to tell. What I have noticed though is that it seems to be helping my vitiligo. I have had only positive side effects so far from the MSM, so I believe I will be able to increase the dosage.

Ms JD, high desert of California, US

I have been on the MSM since April. I go out regularly without a hat, and although I do have makeup on (but no sunscreen), I have not noticed any new patches or darkening. I try to walk 6 miles a day so I am out for some time and the wind up here always blows off my hat! I do avoid, to the best of my ability, being in the sun too long between 10-4pm when the sun is at its strongest, but that is just good common sense for anyone. I do notice some tanning on my face and the darker areas do get a little darker but it all seems to fade at an equal rate.

I'm finally starting to see results with MSM. My chin is almost clear as well as the bridge of my nose. The sides of my nose have lightened a little. My forehead is my trouble spot, it has faded by about 20%, but I do have a few white spots forming in it. I do think if we use common sense we can be in the sun. Nobody wants to sunburn or get aged and wrinkled from deep tanning, so if we use our sunscreen and avoid being in the sun for long periods when the UV's are at their peek, I say why not? We deserve to live a little. Besides studies have shown that getting out in the sun elevates your mood and God knows all us gals could use that, couldn't we?

By the way my cycle has changed from 6-7 days to 2, with no cramping. I used to be at least a week early also, but not anymore. I was 28 days exactly! I feel like I'm finally getting the 'old' me back! I'm 36 and I've known since my last child was born 9 years ago that my hormones have been out of whack, but I couldn't convince a doctor that they were though!

Ms A, Iowa, US

I wanted to share my results with all of you regarding MSM. I have been on it for almost 3 weeks now and feel that I am having great results. I started out taking 9,000 mg per day and currently I'm up to 12,000 mg per day. I did however jump too quickly to 12,000 mg and had to cut back briefly. I was experiencing diarrhea and nagging headaches. I have a weak stomach and it doesn't take much to set it off. But to date, my melasma is fading, my nails are growing like weeds and I could swear that I've lost a few pounds. I'm excited that I've had such good results considering my melasma is the deep kind. I have had several chemical peels, tried all the bleaching creams and consistently use Retin-A (likely always will for its other benefits). My melasma has never budged with any of the above treatments. And if it wasn't for my husband agreeing with my results, I wouldn't believe that MSM is actually working. I'm skeptical to believe in cures that seem too good to be true. But overall it works for me! So, good luck to all of you who are opting to try it!

Abbreviations

BCP = Birth Control Pill

FDA = Food and Drug Administration

GI = Gastro-intestinal

IBS = Irritable Bowel Syndrome

LGS = Leaky Gut Syndrome

RDA = Recommended Daily Amounts

SPF = Sun Protection Factor

UVA/UVB = Ultraviolet A and B rays in sunlight that cause sunburn and skin tanning

A mg (milligram) is one thousandth of a gram (g) - 1 g therefore equals 1000 mg

Glossary

Antioxidant: A substance thought to protect body cells from the damaging effects of oxidation.

Candida: Any of the yeast-like imperfect fungi of the genus Candida that are normally present on the skin and in the mucous membranes of the mouth, intestinal tract and vagina, that may become pathogenic, especially C. albicans; the causative agent of thrush.

Centrofacial: Referring to the central parts of the face, i.e. the 'T-zone'.

Collagen: The fibrous protein constituent of bone, cartilage, tendon and other connective tissue.

Corticosteroid: Any of the steroid hormones produced by the adrenal cortex or their synthetic equivalents, such as cortisol and aldosterone.

Cryotherapy: The local or general use of low temperatures in medical therapy.

Dermis: The sensitive connective tissue layer of the skin located just below the epidermis.

Detoxification: The metabolic process by which the toxic qualities of a poison, chemical or toxin are reduced by or removed from the body.

Elastin: A protein similar to collagen that is the principal structural component of elastic fibres found in body tissues and organs.

Endocrine: Of or relating to endocrine glands or the hormones secreted by them.

Epidermis: The outer protective layer of skin covering the dermis.

Epstein Barr Virus: Is a member of the herpes virus family and one of the most common human viruses. Symptoms include sore throat, swollen lymph glands and chronic fatigue.

Erythema: Redness.

Free radical: A reactive particle that contains an impaired electron making it unstable. Free radicals are encouraged by pollutants such as cigarette smoke and ultraviolet sunlight.

Hyperpigmentation: Excess pigmentation, especially of the skin.

Hypopigmentation: Diminished pigmentation, especially of the skin.

Keratin: A tough, insoluble protein substance that is the chief structural constituent of hair, nails.

Keratinocyte: Skin cell of the keratinised (horny) layer of the epidermis.

Macule: A patch of skin that is discoloured but not usually elevated; caused by various diseases.

Malar: Of or relating to the cheek or the side of the head.

Mandibular: Of the lower jaw.

Melanin: Any of a group of naturally occurring dark pigments, especially the pigment found in skin and hair.

Melanocyte: An epidermal cell capable of synthesising melanin.

Melanogenesis: The formation of melanin.

Menses: The monthly flow of blood and cellular debris from the uterus that begins at puberty in women.

Modality: A therapeutic method or agent, such as surgery, that involves the physical treatment of a disorder.

Pathogen: An agent that causes disease, especially a living micro-organism such as a bacterium or fungus.

Perioral Dermatitis: A condition that generally occurs in the area around the mouth, but it can occur around the nose and (rarely) around the eyes. Symptoms include redness of the skin commonly accompanied by small, sometimes itchy red bumps or even pus bumps, and mild scaling or peeling. In rare cases, a mild burning sensation is experienced.

Peroxidation: The process of peroxidising a chemical compound.

Photosensitive: Sensitive or reactive (sometimes abnormally) to light or other radiant energy.

Pigmentation: Colouring of cells or tissues, e.g. of the skin.

Predisposition: A disposition in advance to react in a particular way.

Propensity: A tendency.

Retinoid: Any of various natural or synthetic derivatives of Vitamin A.

Tinea Versicolor: Tinea Versicolor is a common, benign, superficial cutaneous fungal infection characterised by hypopigmented or hyperpigmented macules that are located primarily on the chest and back. It can, in rare cases, occur on the face. It is not contagious.

Transient: Staying for a short or brief time; not regular or permanent.

Trimester: A period or term of three months.

Tyrosinase: A copper-containing enzyme of plant and animal tissues that catalyses the production of melanin and other pigments from tyrosine by oxidation.

Vitiligo: A rare skin disease consisting of the development of smooth, milk-white spots, which can be surrounded by a heavily pigmented border. It can develop on various parts of the body.

Wood's Lamp: Also known as the 'Black light test' or 'Ultraviolet light test'. This lamp is used to detect bacterial and fungal infections of the skin as well as unusual pigmentary changes, thereby enabling the doctor or dermatologist to gain an insight into the cause of any light or dark coloured spots that are present. The test is performed in a darkened room and the ultraviolet light is shined on the area of interest. It is important to not look at the light during the test.

References

'The Miracle of MSM: The Natural Solution for Pain' by Dr. Stanley W. Jacob MD, Dr. Ronald M. Lawrence MD, PhD, and Martin Zucker, a health writer.

Many other references, pertaining to the 35 years of research carried out by Dr. Stanley W. Jacob, MD, of the Oregon Health Sciences University in Portland Oregon, and Robert Herschler, a research scientist for Crown Zellerbach (who both own the marketing and patent rights to MSM), were sourced from various websites. These are included in the list below of all websites studied in order to gain an understanding of MSM and its general properties prior to writing this book:

www.nutriteam.com/msm.htm
www.msm.com
www.msm-msm.com
www.a1msm.co.uk
www.bulkmsm.com
www.opti-msm.com
www.anewlife.co.uk/msm-candida.html
www.lignisul-msm.com/conditions.html
www.wwns.com/oxygen/msmfacts.htm
www.gowithherbs.com/4059-4.htm

The following websites, alongside various medical dictionaries covering the topics of numerous skin diseases, were referred to in order to gain a greater understanding about melasma and the current treatments available:

www.DrKlein.net
www.dermnetnz.org
www.intelihealth.com
www.ska.safeserver.com

Recommended Reading

'The Miracle of MSM: The Natural Solution for Pain' co-authored by Dr. Stanley W. Jacob MD, Dr. Ronald M. Lawrence MD, PhD, and Martin Zucker, a health writer.